Manual of
CARDIAC SURGERY INSTRUMENTS

Manual of CARDIAC SURGERY INSTRUMENTS

Prashant Shah
MS DNB Cardiac Surgery (Gold Medal)
Head and Sr Consultant
Chief Pediatric and
Congenital Cardiac Surgeon
Kauvery Hospital
Chennai, Tamil Nadu, India

Forewords
MP Naresh Kumar
S Rajan

JAYPEE

JAYPEE BROTHERS MEDICAL PUBLISHERS
The Health Sciences Publisher
New Delhi | London

Jaypee Brothers Medical Publishers (P) Ltd

Headquarters
EMCA House
23/23-B, Ansari Road, Daryaganj
New Delhi 110 002, India
Landline: +91-11-23272143, +91-11-23272703
+91-11-23282021, +91-11-23245672
E-mail: jaypee@jaypeebrothers.com

Corporate Office
4838/24, Ansari Road, Daryaganj
New Delhi 110 002, India
Phone: +91-11-43574357
Fax: +91-11-43574314
E-mail: jaypee@jaypeebrothers.com

Overseas Office
J.P. Medical Ltd
83 Victoria Street, London
SW1H 0HW (UK)
Phone: +44 20 3170 8910
E-mail: info@jpmedpub.com

EU GPSR Authorised Representative
Logos Europe, 9 rue Nicolas Poussin
17000, La Rochelle, France
Phone: +33 (0) 6 67 93 73 78
E-mail: contact@logoseurope.eu

Website: www.jaypeebrothers.com
Website: www.jaypeedigital.com

Inquiries for bulk sales may be solicited at: jaypee@jaypeebrothers.com

Manual of Cardiac Surgery Instruments

First Edition: 2016

Reprint: 2026

ISBN: 978-93-5250-006-2

Printed in India

Dedicated to

All my teachers
Dr KM Cherian, Dr S Rajan,
Dr Robert Coelho and Dr VM Kurian
from whom I have learned my basics of cardiac surgery

Foreword

Human race is a tool using primate species and the only one capable of devising tools to perform and enhance its motor activities and sensory inputs.

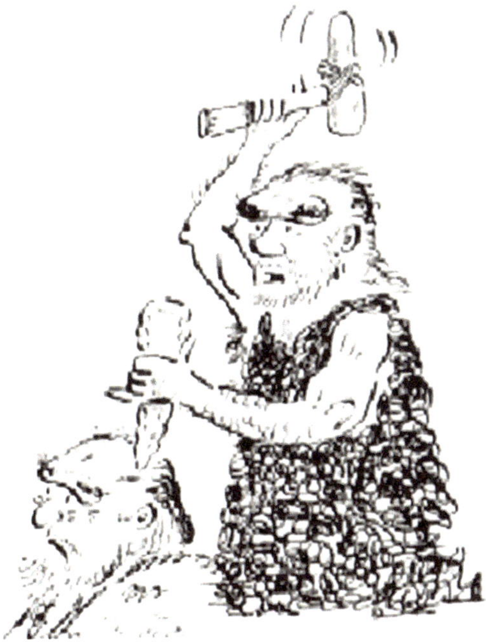

Surgical tools have been existing from the early history of mankind.

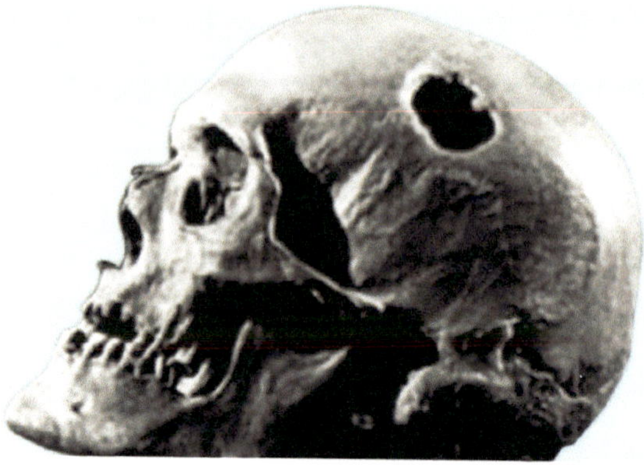

"It is even probable that the trephine holes found in prehistoric skull of 50,000 years old were made for curative purposes."

—Professor Kappers

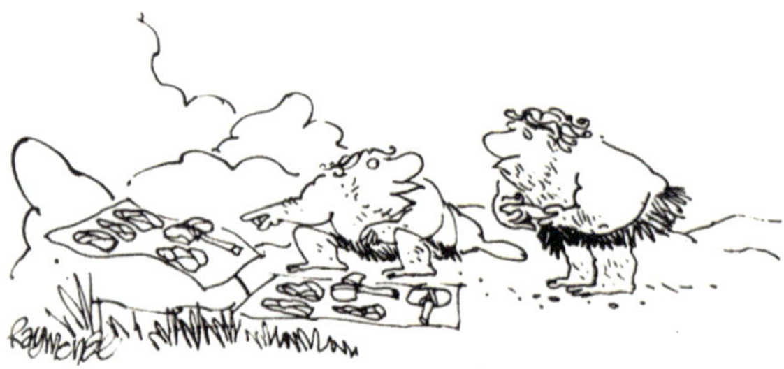

"Naturally they're more expensive—they're surgical instruments."

It is no wonder that the tools of trade for cardiac surgery and cardiology, which is the culmination of almost all disciplines in the field of healing, require the very best.

The growth and development in the field of cardiac surgery happens to coincide happily with an era of technological development never seen before in human history, and this has led to a quantum leap in surgical tool making, particularly in the field of cardiology and cardiac surgery.

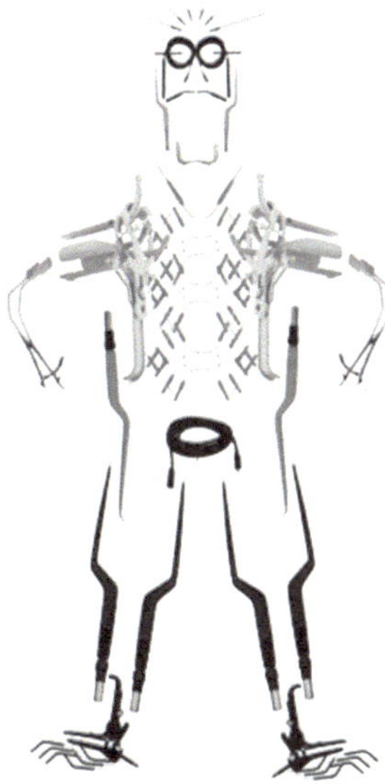

The modern tools of cardiac surgery have not only made it possible to perform complex operations from arterial switches to heart transplantation but also made these very safe for the patients.

I congratulate Dr Shah, for trying to compile the *Manual of Cardiac Surgery Instruments* to appraise its practitioners as to the variety of tools available and how they were developed.

The book would be a very useful tool for students of surgery, particularly cardiac surgery and also paramedical staff and nursing staff.

MP Naresh Kumar
MS MCh FRCS FICS FIACS DSc (Hon)
Head and Sr Consultant Cardiac Surgeon
Harvey Cardiac Centre
Chennai, Tamil Nadu, India

Foreword

It gives me immense pleasure and pride to write the foreword for this book titled, *Manual of Cardiac Surgery Instruments*, written by Dr Prashant Shah. He was my student in Diplomate of National Board (DNB) at Institute of Cardiovascular Diseases (ICVD), Madras Medical Mission. Prashant Shah was very studious and a talented student. He was awarded the Gold Medal by the National Board for his brilliant work.

Throughout his training, he remained one of the finest human beings—always respecting and loving others. His communication with patients was sensitive and caring. This communication and expressive skill has blossomed in the way of creating this book. I can foresee that all these wonderful qualities will take him to greater heights and enable him to achieve more in life.

I am sure this book will be of great use to everyone in the field of cardiac surgery, especially to the students and trainees while they are learning and putting their conceptual knowledge into practical use. Great amount of time and effort has gone into making this book, and I sincerely hope this will be read by many and promoted widely.

I wish Prashant Shah happiness and success in all his endeavors, and a very bright future in his academics as well as in clinical practice.

S Rajan MS MCh
Head and Director
Department of Cardiac Surgery
Madras Medical Mission
Chennai, Tamil Nadu, India
Secretary
Indian Association of Cardiothoracic Surgeons

Preface

Cardiac surgeons are like warriors who fight against disease with their instruments.

Instruments are basic necessities for any type of surgery.

Right instrument at right place makes surgery safe and simple.

Along with general surgery instruments, there are different types of instruments available for use in cardiac surgery.

In the early part of my training in cardiac surgery and while preparing for my examinations, I had to struggle to learn features and use of different instruments used in cardiac surgery. I started collecting facts on the commonly used instruments. This book is a byproduct of that work.

I hope this book will serve as a good companion for trainee cardiac surgeons, cardiac theater nurses and paramedical staff.

I wish all the best to the readers.

Prashant Shah

Acknowledgments

To build this book, it took me nearly a year and there are good number of people who helped me directly or indirectly in this project.

I acknowledge Dr Sanjay Theodore and Dr MM Yusuf for their contribution in Chapter 11, Mr Paneer Selvam for Chapter 12, Ms Jayanthi and Mr Jayshankar for Chapters 13, 14 and 15.

I am grateful to Dr S Rajan and Dr MP Naresh Kumar, for their guidance and excellent foreword for this book.

I thank Mr Ritesh Hebbar from Hebbar Surgical, Mr Siva Kumar—Centenial Sutures and Mr Vijay Kumar—Lotus Sutures, for their kind support.

I acknowledge Medtronic Inc and Maque Inc, for granting permission to use photographs of their products.

I thank Shri Jitendar P Vij (Group Chairman), Mr Ankit Vij (Group President) and Mr Tarun Duneja (Director-Publishing) and the team of M/s Jaypee Brothers Medical Publishers (P) Ltd, New Delhi, India, for their excellent work and cooperation.

Contents

CHAPTER 1

Sternal Saw

Sternal saw is a bone cutter, introduced by Dr Edward B Diethrich in 1963.[1]

TYPES

Sternal saw is of two types:

a. Reciprocating
b. Oscillatory

Uses: Median sternotomy and partial sternotomy.

Reciprocal Saw

Different types of reciprocating blade saw are available.

Hand Operating Type

In hand operating, operating lever is situated in handpiece only
Easy to use, no other connection requires
Easy to maintain
Battery operated so charging require before use

Foot Operating Type

- Handpiece is connected to driving unit with special cable
- Cheaper in cost

- Heavy to use
- Cable connection to handpiece makes it difficult to use in certain position (Fig. 1.1)

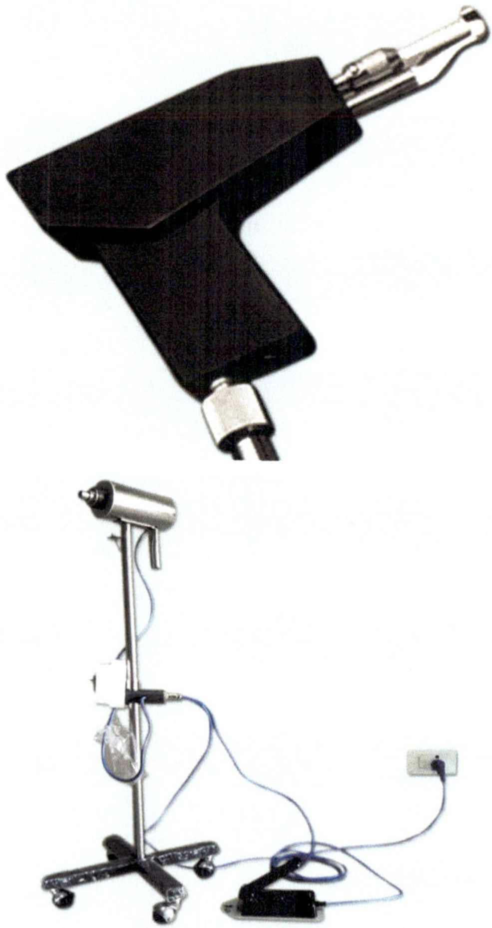

A

B

Fig. 1.1: Reciprocal saw

Oscillatory Type

- Different models of oscillatory type of saw available
- Battery operated models (Fig. 1.2).
- Handpiece has a switch to operate the saw.
- Different sizes of blades available, according to size of the patient we have to change blade.

Foot Operated Models

- This model has three parts, driving unit, handpiece and blade (Fig. 1.3).

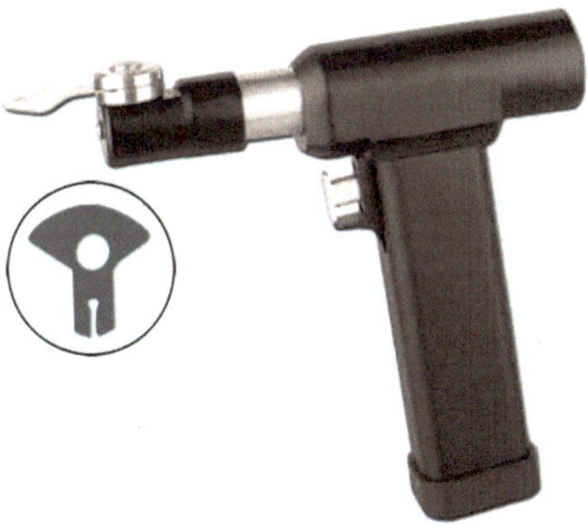

Fig. 1.2: Battery-operated oscillatory saw

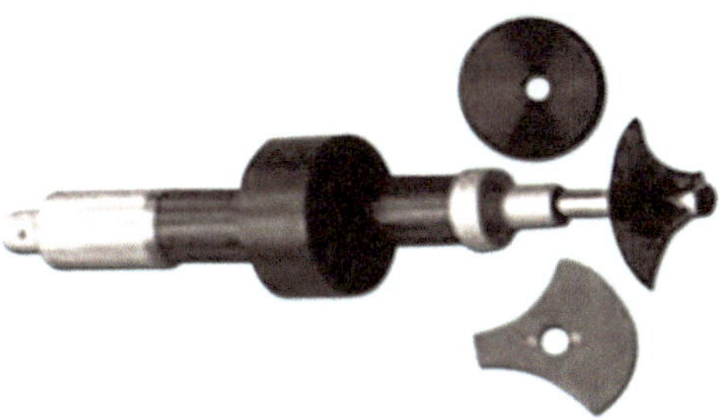

Fig. 1.3: Foot operated model

- With special cable hand piece is connected to driving unit which runs by electric current.
- Different models are available.

Use

- Redo sternotomy
- Neonates and infant sternotomy
- Partial sternotomy.

Q. What are the care you should take during sternotomy?

- During dissection at suprasternal notch dissection should be over the sternum dissecting carelessly at this place can injure innominate artery or vein
- In aortic stenosis with dilated ascending aorta you should be more careful
- Dissection at subxiphoid region. Make a plane between sternum and pericardium with blunt dissection with finger or artery forceps. This space will help to engage the sternal head where you can do down to up sternotomy.

Q. Why you should keep lung down during sternotomy?

- It will provide space between sternum and pericardium
- Injury to pleural can be avoided
- During expiration heart has a small volume so size of heart is smaller.

Q. What are the other ways to do sternotomy?

Giglee wire saw can be used (Fig. 1.4).

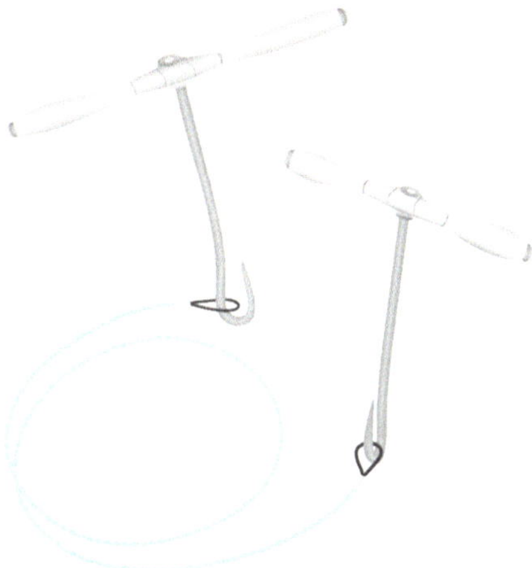

Fig. 1.4: Giglee wire saw

Method

- After creating plane at suprasternal notch and subxiphoid region pass giglee wire from top to bottom
- Keep open gauze piece below wire
- Sawing movement will cut sternum

LEBSCHE STERNAL KNIFE (FIG. 1.5)

Mayo scissors for small babies.

Q. What are the care you should take during redo sternotomy?

- Keep access for femoral cannulation
- Do gentle dissection through subxiphoid region and make a place between heart and sternum
- Dissection under vision
- Keep lower pressure and lungs down during sternotomy
- Lift the sternum by sternal wires or catspaw

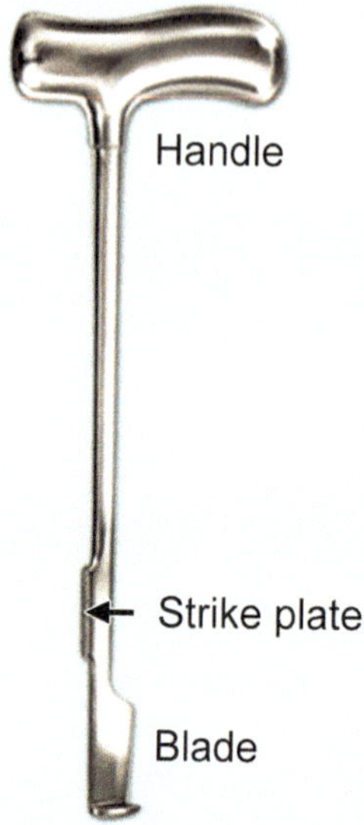

Fig. 1.5: Lebsche sternal knife

- Use oscillatory saw and cut up to inner table step by step and proceed further up
- Pre-operative X-ray chest lateral view will guide you which place you should be careful
- Situation where calcified conduit or aorta stuck to sternum elective femorofemoral bypass will help to decompress the heart.

REFERENCES

1. Surgery.1963 12 01 sternal saw—new instrument for splitting the sternum. DIETHRICH EB, MORRIS JD. Surgery.PMID14027806

CHAPTER

2

Clamps

HISTORY

First development of atraumatic forceps, which facilitate vascular reconstruction by temporarily clamping vessels was by Edmund Hopfner in 1903 at the Berlin University Hospital.[1]

The first tangential occlusion clamp was developed by Friedrich Trendelenburg in 1908, when he established the operative treatment for embolism of the pulmonary artery. This clamp was later modified by AW Meyer and VP Satinsky.

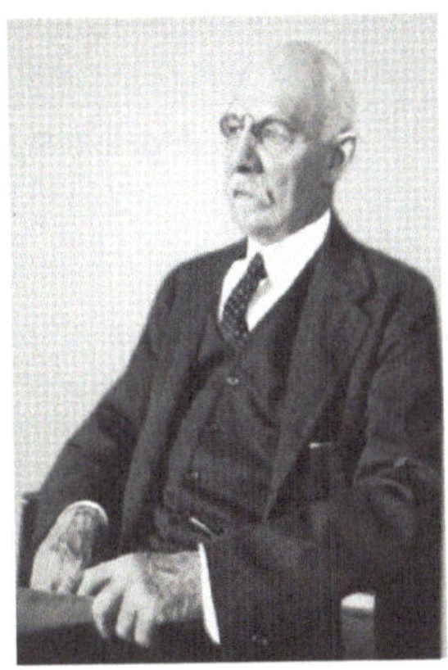

Fig. 2.1: William Stewart Halsted (1852–1922)

William Stewart Halsted (1852–1922)

William stewart Halsted was the first to ligate and excise subclavian aneurysm (1892) and to pioneer attempts to manage abdominal aortic aneurysm by proximal banding (Fig. 2.1).[2,3]

He developed halsted clamp as prior clamps were crude and traumatic on vessels.

Michael E. DeBakey (1908–2008)

Michael E DeBakey (Fig. 2.2) is one of the greatest surgeon innovators in cardiac surgery. He developed roller pump for heart lung machine. He developed and pioneered the use of Dacron grafts for repair of aorta, atraumatic vascular clamps and forceps.[4-8]

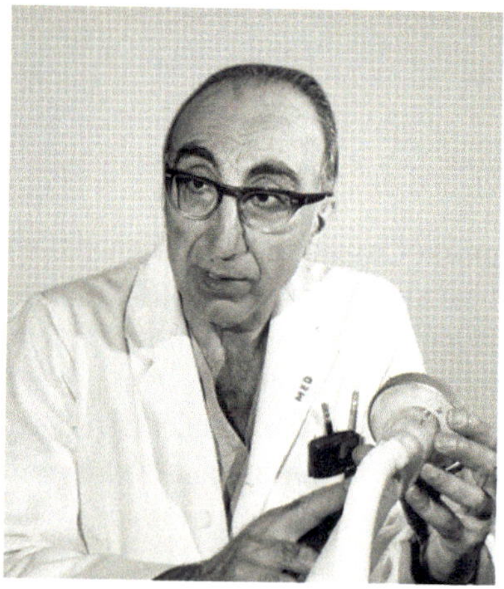

Fig. 2.2: Michael E. Debakey (1908-2008)

Victor P Satinsky (1912-1997)

As a research director at Hahnemann Cardiovascular Institute Philadelphia, Victor P Satinsky developed at least 30 major medical innovations. Satinsky vascular clamp is still widely used today.[9,10]

Denton Cooley

Denton Colley (Fig. 2.3) revolutionized the field of cardiac surgery by developing surgical technique to treat aortic

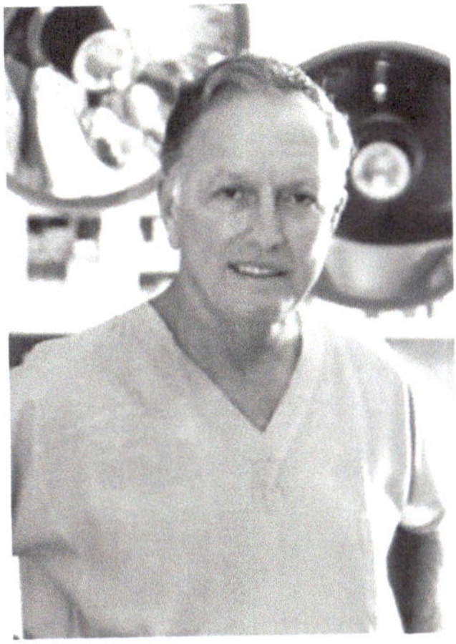

Fig. 2.3: Denton Cooley

aneurysm, to modernize the cardiopulmonary bypass machine and to conceive the first left ventricular assist device. He developed several atraumatic vascular clamps and forceps which are still in use across the world.[5]

Ernest Stanley Crawford (1922–1992)

One of the DeBakey's students, Earnes stanley crawford developed innovative surgical techniques for the management of aortic dissection and complex aortic diseases. Crawford aortic clamps are frequently used in surgical theaters today.[11]

VASCULAR CLAMPS

- Ideal vascular clamp occlude the vessel lumen and protect intima and wall of vessel
- Vascular clamps are differentiated by its shape and serrations
- Different shapes and angled clamps are available for use at different site.

Serrations Type

It is described in Chapter 4 (Figs 4.12 and 4.13, page 51).

DeBakey's Type

- DeBakey's type has two rows of finely serrated teeth on one side of blade and one on opposing blade.

Cooley's Type

- Cooley's type blade has a double raw (2 × 2) of finally serrated teeth on both side.

Castaneda Type

- Single row of fine serrations which are precisely meshed.

2 × 3 Vascular Teeth

- This type has three rows of finely serrated teeth on one blade and two rows on the opposing blade (Fig. 2.4).

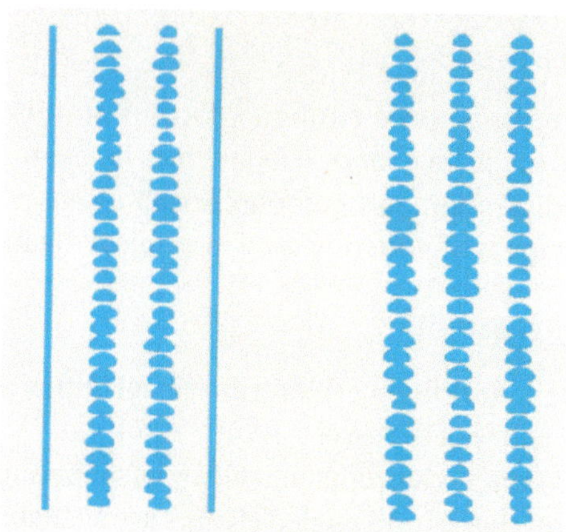

Fig. 2.4: 2 × 3 vascular teeth

Advantage

- Better occlusion
- Secure grasp of tissue.

TYPES OF VASCULAR CLAMPS

Cross Clamps

- These clamps are used for total occlusion of a vessel.
- It is available in straight, curved, obtuse angle, and right angle (Fig. 2.5).

Partial Occlusion Clamp

- This clamp is used for the occlusion of a portion of a vessel or chamber and permitting continuous flow of blood into native vessel (Fig. 2.5).

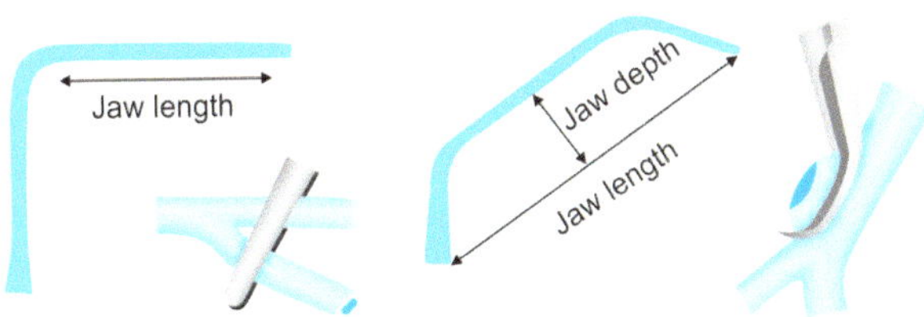

Fig. 2.5: Cross clamp and partial occlusion clamp

Cooley's Vascular Clamp

- Identification through pattern of serrations and marks on inner aspect of clamp. Cooley's type cross clamps and partial occlusion clamps as shown in Figure 2.6.

Uses

- Clamping right atrial appendage for purse-string
- Clamping LA appendage for occlusion

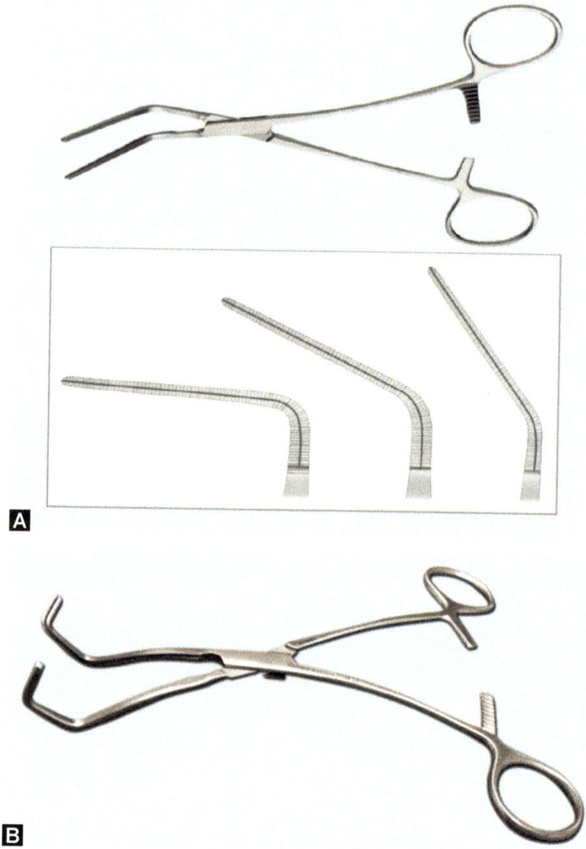

Fig. 2.6: Cooley's clamps

- BT shunt, central shunt at aortic and pulmonary end
- Aortic cannulation
- Proximal graft anastomosis in CABG.
- Partial clamping of pulmonary artery in Glenn and Fontan surgery

- PDA clamping for division and suturing
- Cross clamp uses are described in DeBakey's clamp uses.

DeBakey Clamp

- Identification by peculiar 1 × 2 serration
- Any size and shape available
- Combination of diffrent clamp with DeBakey serrations are available
- Atraumatic and does not come in surgical field
- Crest present beyond the jaw of the clamp for accommodating arterial wall to avoid puckering (Fig. 2.7).

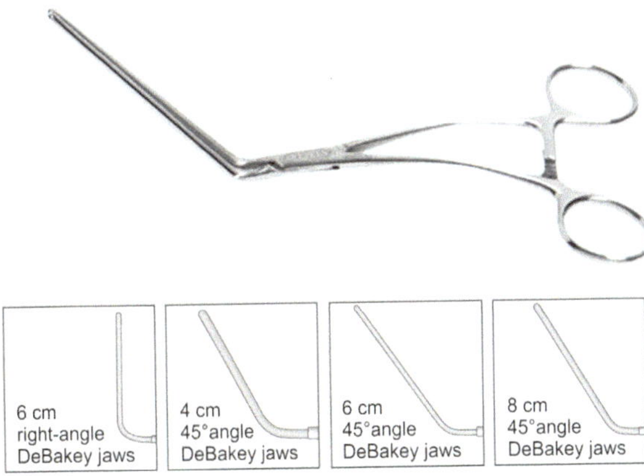

Fig. 2.7: DeBakey's clamp

Uses

- Cross clamping of aorta in open heart surgery
- Clamping of PDA
- Clamping of IVC during Fontan surgery
- Clamping of aorta in aneurysm surgery
- Peripheral vascular surgery to clamp vessel.

Castaneda Vascular Clamp

- Identification through serration pattern
- Different size, shape and angulation available (Fig. 2.8).

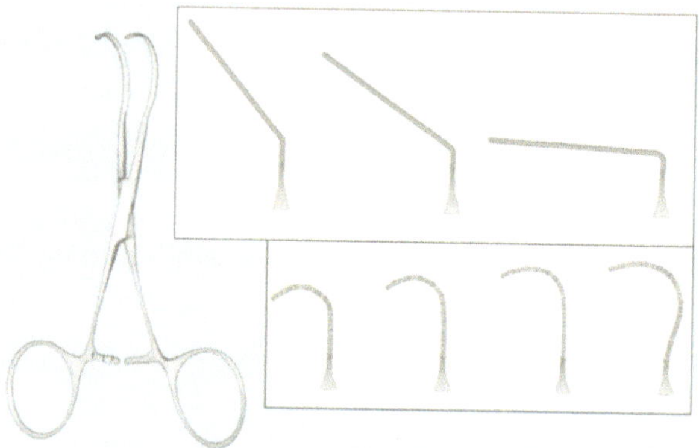

Fig. 2.8: Castaneda vascular clamp

Uses

Same like DeBakey and Cooley's clamp.

Derra Clamp

- Partial occlusion clamp (Fig. 2.9)
- Jaw depth is larger than Cooley's clamp.

Uses

- Fontan procedure to clamp pulmonary artery partially
- Proximal anastomosed in CABG.

Satinsky Clamp

- Identification (Fig. 2.10).

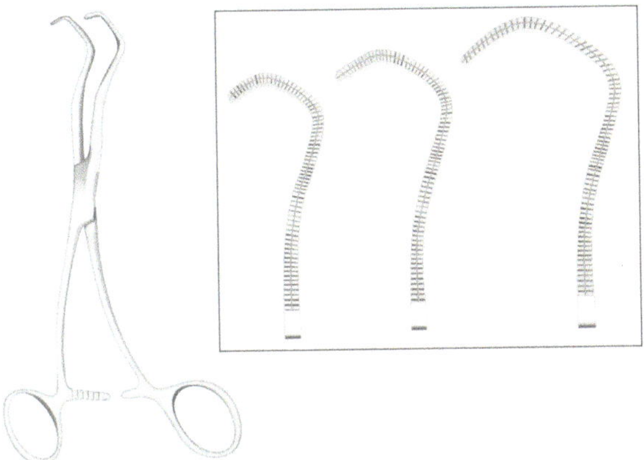

Fig. 2.9: Derra clamp

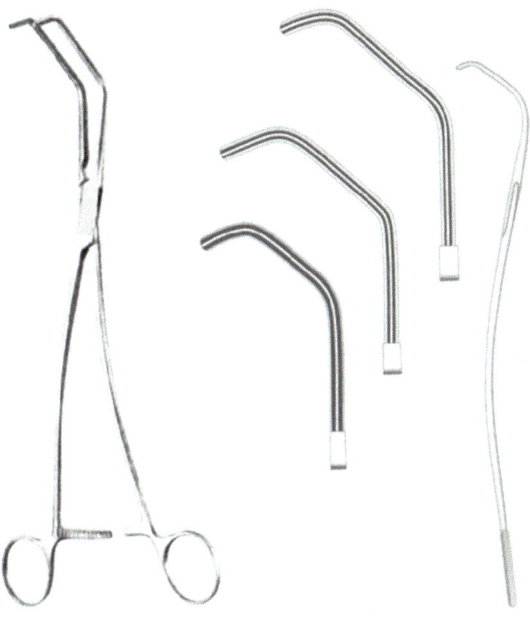

Fig. 2.10: Satinsky clamp

- Different jaw depth is available
- Serrations are DeBakey's type.

Uses

- Side bitting of aorta during proximal anastomosis in CABG
- Encircling of IVC
- Clamping of LA appendage during closed mitral commissurotomy
- Waldehausen repair for coarctation
- Other same as Cooley's clamp uses.

Lambert-Kay Aorta Partial Occlusion Clamp

- Identification point (Fig. 2.11):
  Serration DeBakey's type
  Augulation in body
  Blade Satinsky type.

Use

Same like Satinsky clamp.

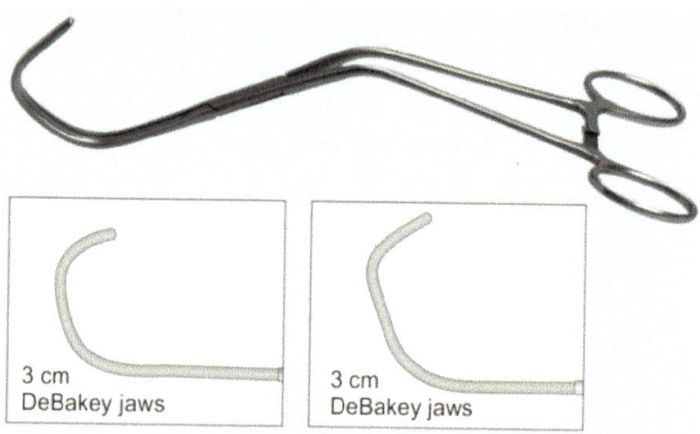

Fig. 2.11: Lambert-Kay aorta partial occlusion clamp

Bulldog Clamp

Gregory Classic Bulldog Clamps (Fig. 2.12)

- 1 × 2 type DeBakey serration
- Straight and angle jaw
- Different sizes available.

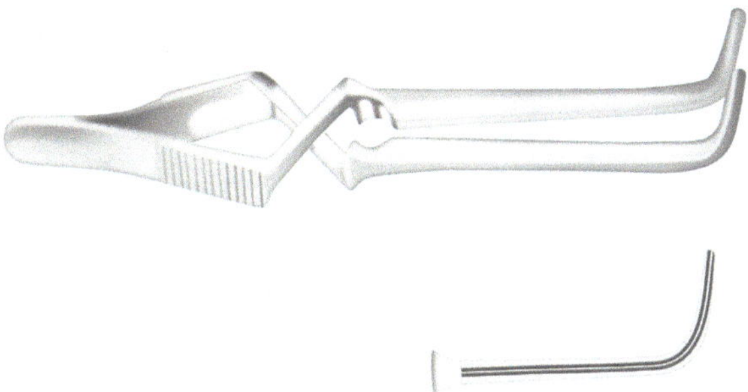

Fig. 2.12: Gregory classic bulldog clamps

Diethrich Bulldog Clamps

- Smaller jaw length (Fig. 2.13)

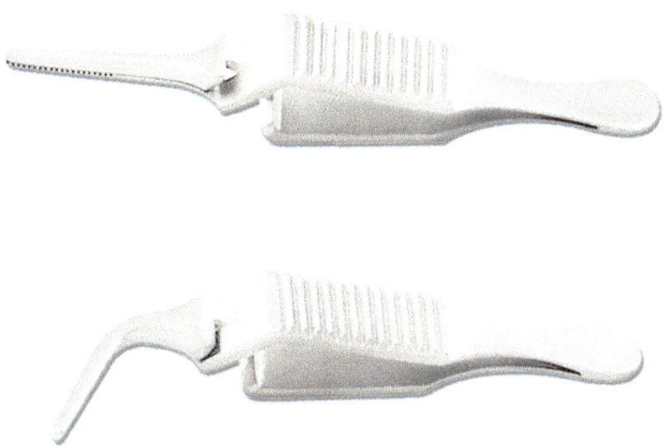

Fig. 2.13: Diethrich bulldog clamps

- Nonserrated jaw
- Tension 22 g and modified tension bulldog (180 g).

Glover Classic Bulldog Clamp

- Serration type 1 × 2 vascular teeth (Fig. 2.14)
- Different jaw teeth and body teeth available

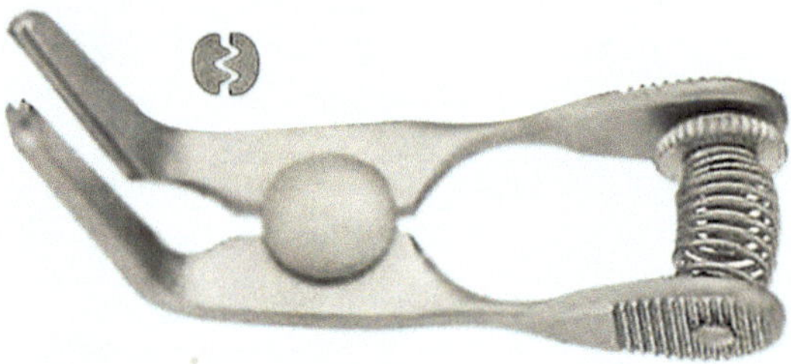

Fig. 2.14: Glover classic bulldog clamp

Jacobson Bulldog

- Serrated jaw simple
- Curved and straight (Fig. 2.15).

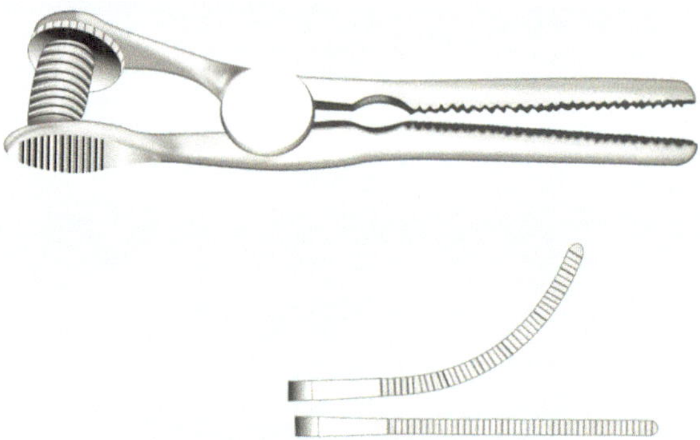

Fig. 2.15: Jacobson bulldog clamp

Uses of Bulldog

- Clamping of small blood vessel
- Clamping of IMA after its division (Less tension soft bulldog should be used)
- Clamping of venous graft after distal anastomosis
- Holding sutures (nonserrated is ideal or cover serration with soft rubber)
- During Atrioveneous fistula creation to clamp artery and vein.

Vorse–Webster Tube Occluding Clamp

- Tough instruments (Fig. 2.16)
- Guard at joint level to give support to blade
- Transverse course serrations.

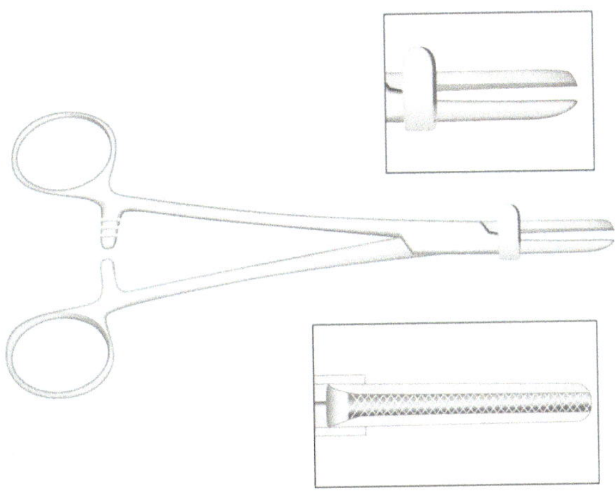

Fig. 2.16: Vorse–Webster tube occluding clamp

Uses

- Clamping of tubes for division before going on bypass
- Clamping of aortic cannula, post-insertion for deairing and checking pulsaltile flow
- Clamping of venous cannula when on bypass with single cannula
- Clamping of venous cannula for coming off bypass
- Intercostal drainage tube clamp.

Q. Which surgeries on CPB can be performed without aortic cross clamping?

- BDG, extracardiac Fontan procedure
- Pulmonary valvotomy
- Right sided tumor excision
- Tricuspid valve procedure
- CABG.

Q. What are the other ways of cross-clamping aorta?

- Endoluminal balloon occlusion for port access surgery and calcified, atheromatous aorta [TEE guidance require to place above coronary arteries and aortic valve]

Q. Which conditions require early clamping of aorta?

- Aortic regurgitation
- Truncus arteriosus
- AP window
- Myxoma.

Q. What are the complications of aortic cross-clamp?

- Clamp may be applied partially which may leak blood and cardioplegia may not be effective

- Improper aortic cross-clamp can block left main coronary artery can lead to left sided ischemia
- Tip of cardioplegia cannula can come in clamp
- Damage intima and cause dissection of Aorta
- Dislodgement of plaque cause embolic event
- Rupture of aortic wall.

Q. What care you should take during aortic cross clamp?

- Check aorta for atheroma or calcification and choose proper site
- Reduce the flow to minimum so aorta will be soft
- Check the tip of aortic cross clamp which should be beyond aorta
- Make sure of aortic cannula and cardioplegia cannula tip.

Q. Why should we reduce flow during declamping of aorta?

- On clamped aorta, aortic valve cusps are open and on release of the clamp blood may gush to LV and distend it. So to prevent LV distension flow should be reduced and declamp the aorta.

REFERENCES

1. World j Surg. 1998 May;22(5):499-505.
2. Cameron JL. William Stewart Halsted: our surgical heritage. Ann Surg. 1997;225:445-58.
3. Burjet WC. Surgical papers by William Stewart Halsted. Johns Hopkins Press, Baltimore. MD;1924
4. DeBakey surgical innovations. Baylor College of Medicine. www.bcm.edu/news/packages/medinnovations.cfm
5. DeBakey ME, Cooley DA, Crawford ES, et al. Clinical application of a new flexible knitted Dacron arterial substitute. Am Surg. 1958;24:861-9.

6. Mitka M, DeBakey ME. Father of modern cardiac surgery. JAMA. 2005;293:913-8.
7. Sorelle R. Milestone for Dr Debakey. Circulation 1998;98:1255-6.
8. DeBakey ME. Health care hall of fame. Mod healthc. 1996;26:22-4.
9. Eisen Md, Brayman KL, Satinsky VP. Victor Satinsky and success of his partially occluding vascular clamp. Trans stud coll Physicians Phila. 2000;22:87-104.
10. Satinsky MA, Satinsky VP. Victor Paul Satinsky-renaissance doc. Curr surg. 2004,61:402-3.
11. Crawford ES. www.debakeydepartmentofsurgery.org/home/content (content id-289)

CHAPTER

3

Retractors

HISTORY

Theodore Tuffier (1857–1929)

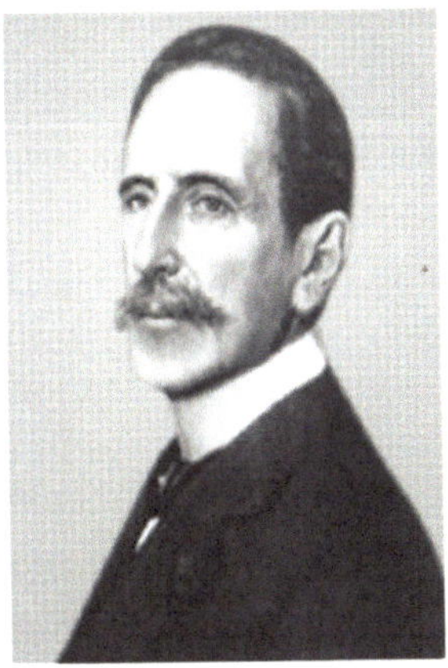

Fig. 3.1: Theodore Tuffier (1857–1929)

Theodore Tuffier (1857-1929) (Fig. 3.1) a French surgeon and pioneer, introduced his first rack and pinion retractor during World War I.

Later simple screw was added at John Hopkins hospital so that instrument stays in desired position. Today, there are many version of Tuffier retractor but the inspiration of Tuffier and his foray into thoracic cavity allowed the further advancement of thoracic and cardiovascular surgery.[1]

Enrique Finochietto (1881–1948)

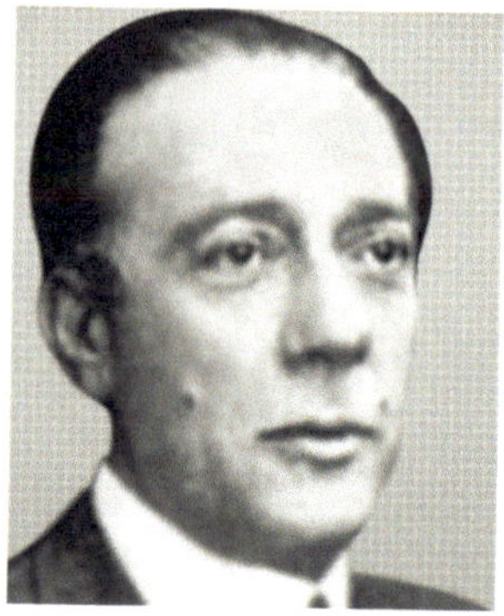

Fig. 3.2: Enrique Finochietto (1881–1948)

Enrique Finochietto (1881-1948) (Fig. 3.2) an Argentinian surgeon, great surgeon innovator, a hero among his people and decorated ambassador of surgery. During 1920 he developed more than 67 different instruments, including thoracic rib retractor, a hand drill and electrically motorized surgical table.[2,3]

- Retractors are made for good exposure of the operation filed
- Proper retractor should be used at correct site and angle with proper traction to avoid damage to tissue due to traction and compression.

TYPES OF RETRACTOR

- Hand-held (plain) retractors
- Self-retaining retractors.

HAND-HELD PLAIN RETRACTOR

- This is a simple instrument with blade on one or either side
- Commonly used plain retractors in cardiac surgery are mentioned below.

Langenbeck Retractor

- This is a commonly used retractor
- Small blade and larger blade sizes are available (Fig. 3.3).

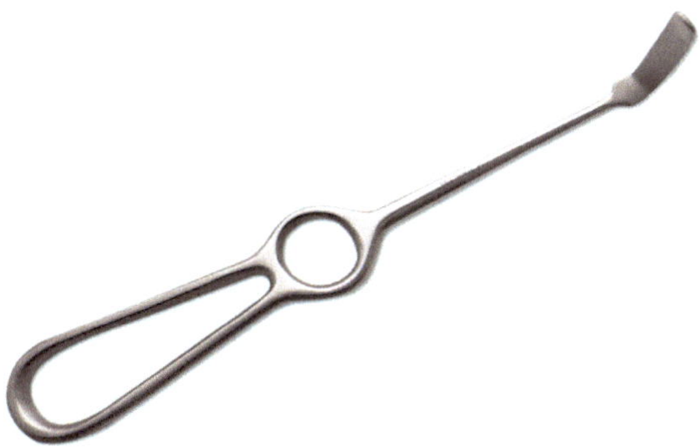

Fig. 3.3: Langenbeck retractor

Uses

- During suprasternal notch and subxiphoid area dissection
- After sternotomy to retract sternum for hemostasis
- Retract sternum after sternal wiring to see wire site bleeding
- Ministernotomy case for better exposure
- Retracting RA or LA for valve procedure.

Davidson Scapula Retractor

- Larger blade helps to support scapula while space between blade and handle helps to accommodate muscle tissue
- Good hand grip helps assistant (Fig. 3.4).

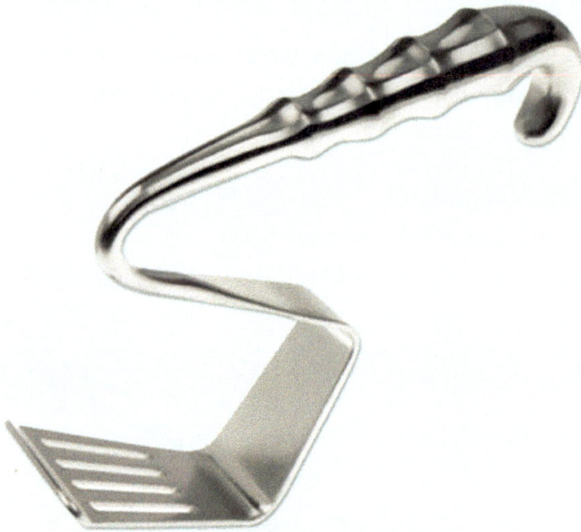

Fig. 3.4: Davidson scapula retractor

Uses

- In all lateral and posterolateral thoracotomy procedure, scapula retraction requires intercostal space identification and incision.

Allison Lung Retractors

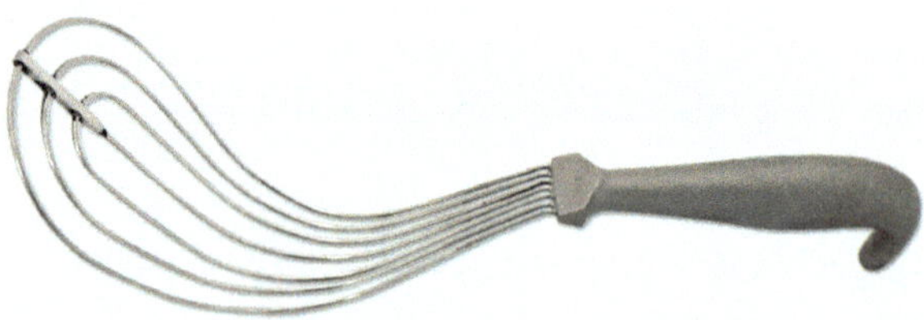

Fig. 3.5: Allison lung retractors

Uses

- Retraction of lung during Lobectomy
- PDA ligation, coarctation of aorta repair, BT shunt surgery
- Thoracotomy ASD closure, mitral valve repair (Fig. 3.5).

Cooley's Atrial Retractor

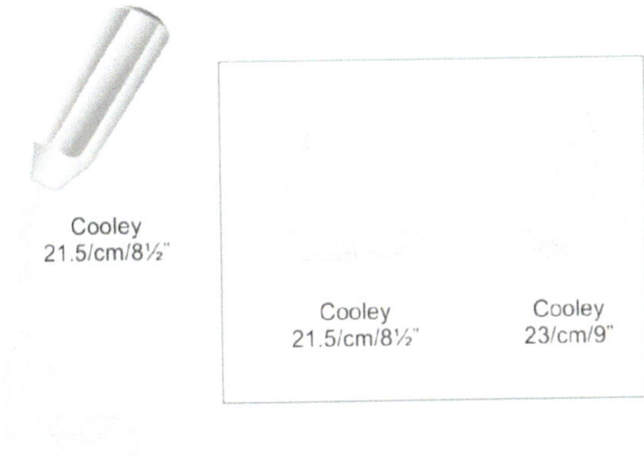

Fig. 3.6: Cooley's atrial retractor

Identification

- This retractor has angulation at 2 places
- First angulation at handle side and other at blade side
- Shape of blade kept in such a way that during retraction it accommodates tissue (Fig. 3.6)
- Connecting curved wire has multiple serrations for better grip of tissue.

Uses

- Mitral valve repair and replacement for LA retraction
- LA myxoma removal
- Atrial fibrillation surgery.

Modification—Modified retractor without handle for self-retaining retractor available.

Kirklin Atrial Retractors

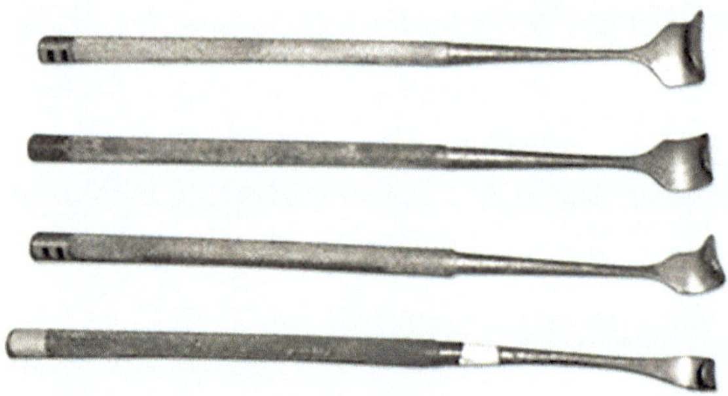

Fig. 3.7: Kirklin atrial retractors

Identification

- Small curved blade with long shaft
- Different size of blades are available (Fig. 3.7).

Uses

- Retraction of right atrium for ASD closure.
- Retraction of tricuspid valve leaflet for infundibular resection and VSD closure
- Retraction of pulmonary valve during transpulmonary VSD closure and resection
- Retraction of aortic valve for septal myomectomy
- Aortic valve replacement for aortic wall retraction.

Liddicoat Aortic Valve Retractor

- Curved blade with side to side curvature (Fig. 3.8).

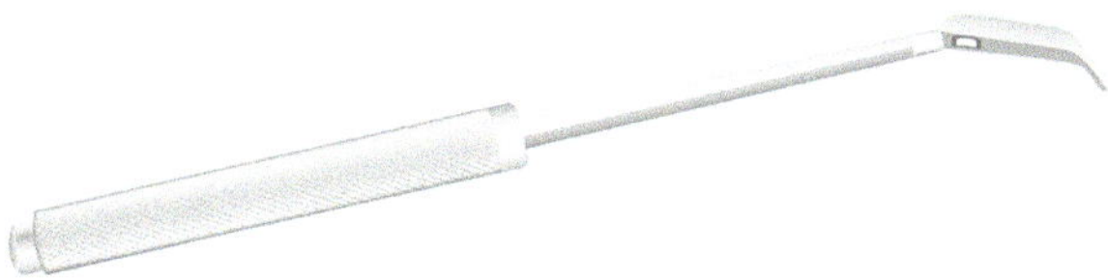

Fig. 3.8: Liddicoat retractor

Uses

- Aortic valve repair and replacement
- Aortic valve retraction in—
  - Subaortic membrane resection
  - Subaortic VSD closure
  - HOCM—septal myomectomy.

CRILE Hook Retractor

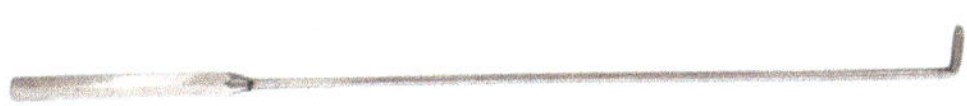

Fig. 3.9: Crile hook retractor

- Tip
  - Sharp tip or
  - Ball tip.

Uses

- Retraction of chordae in mitral valve repair.

Malleable Retractor

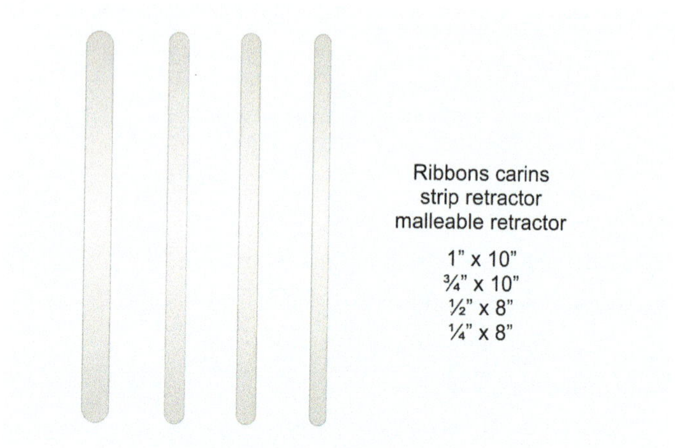

Fig. 3.10: Malleable retractors

Thin round edge malleable strips of metal. Different sizes available (Fig. 3.10).

Uses

- RVOT resection for retraction of tricuspid valve
- Transinfundibular VSD closure
- Subaortic membrane resection
- Transpulmonary muscle resection.

Cat's Paw Retractor

Identification

- This is a biblade instrument with one side 3 curved prongs while other side curved small blade like langenback (Fig. 3.11).

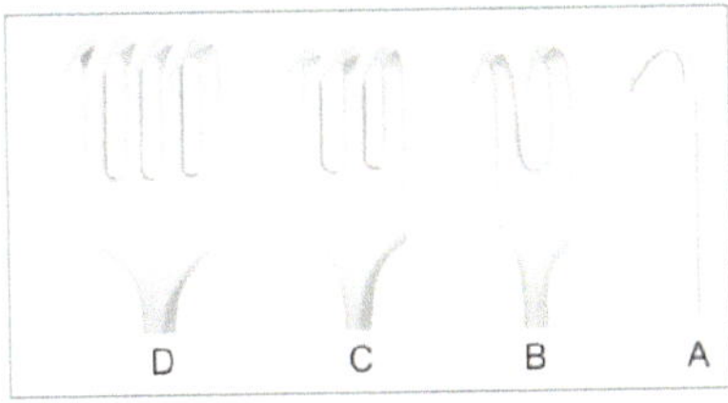

Fig. 3.11: Cat's paw retractor

Uses

- Retraction of suprasternal notch for dissection during sternotomy
- Retraction of sternum in babies
- Redo sternotomy to retract lower part of the sternum.

Rake Retractor

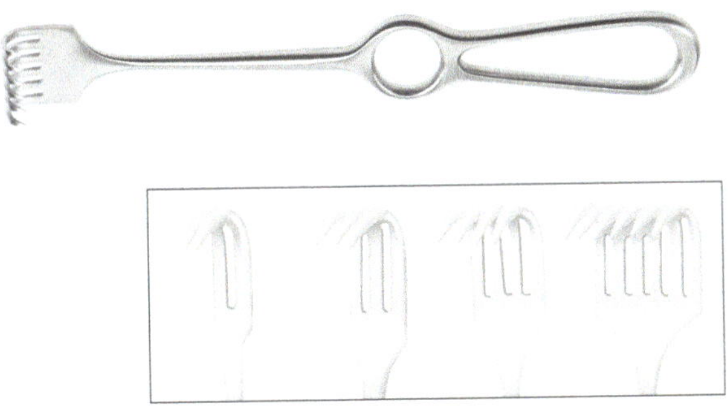

Fig. 3.12: Rake retractor

Identification

- Two or multiple curved prongs in blade while handle has a finger grip in center and palm grip (Fig. 3.12).

Uses

- Retraction of sternum during redo sternotomy
- Lifting of sternum during use of oscillatory saw
- Subxiphoid tissue retraction.

Murphy Retractor

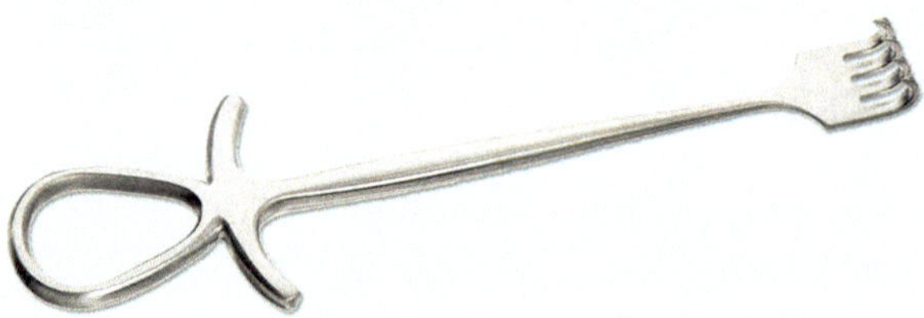

Fig. 3.13: Murphy retractor

- Same like rake retractor only handle is different (Fig. 3.13).

Ross Retractor

Identification

- Right-angled curved blade differentiation from Liddicoat aortic valve retractor
- Right-angled blade
- Handle and shaft is different (Fig. 3.14).

Uses

- Same like Liddicoat aortic valve retractor.

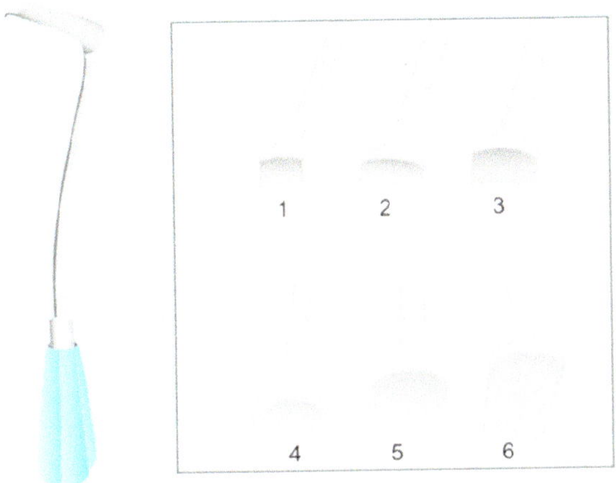

Fig. 3.14: Ross' aortic retractor 9' 228 mm

SELF RETAINING RETRACTORS

Sternal Retractors

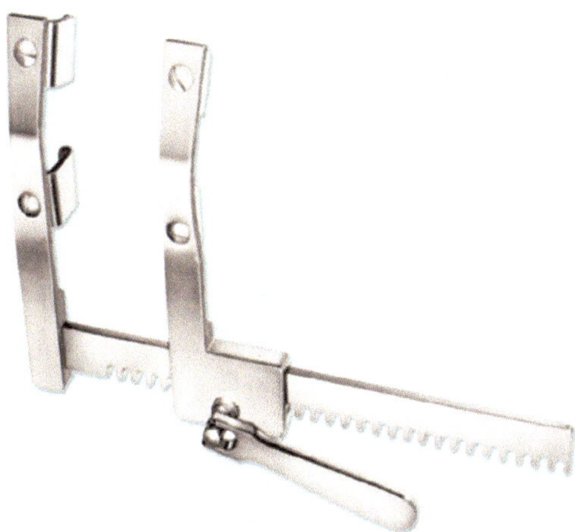

Fig. 3.15: Morse sternal retractor

Morse Sternal Retractor

- Rack and pinion action with mobile sternal blade
- Pediatric and adult size available
- In Favaloro modification sternal blades are fixed (Fig. 3.15).

Uses

- Sternal retraction after median sternotomy
- Pinion and rank can be positioned either toward the patient heart or at subcostal area

Ankeney Sternal Retractor

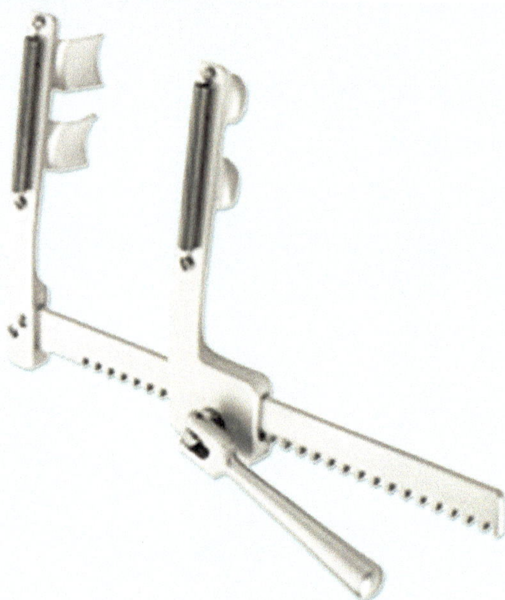

Fig. 3.16: Ankeney sternal retractor

- Rack and pinion action
- Body of aluminium while rack stainless steel
- Four fixed swivel blades (Fig. 3.16).

Advantage

- Due to aluminium, light reflection can be avoided
- Light weight.

Modification

- Three rows of detachable blades on either sides (Fig. 3.17).

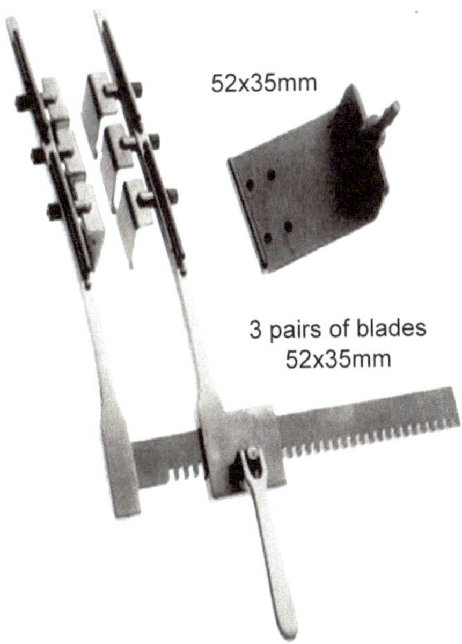

Fig. 3.17: Modification over ankenay's retractor

Castaneda Infant Sternal Retractor

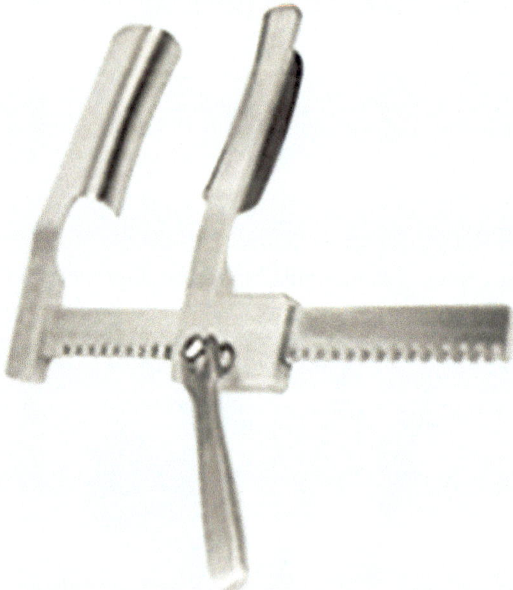

Fig. 3.18: Castaneda infant sternal retractor

- Rack and pinion action
- Aluminum small blade with curvature (Fig. 3.18)
- Rack is stainless steel.

Advantage

- Better sternal grip
- Curvature gives good lateral exposure
- Light weight.

Collins Sternal Retractors

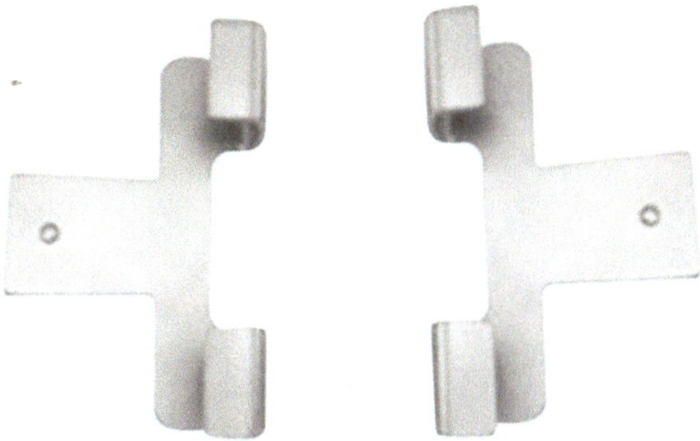

A

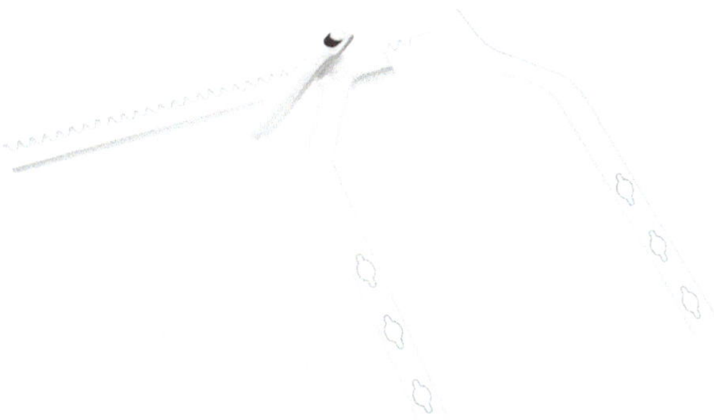

B

Figs 3.19A and B: Collins sternal retractors

- Body and blades are separate
- Different size of blades available that can be chosen according to the size of the patient (Fig. 3.19)
- Steel and plastic blades available.

Carpentier Retractor

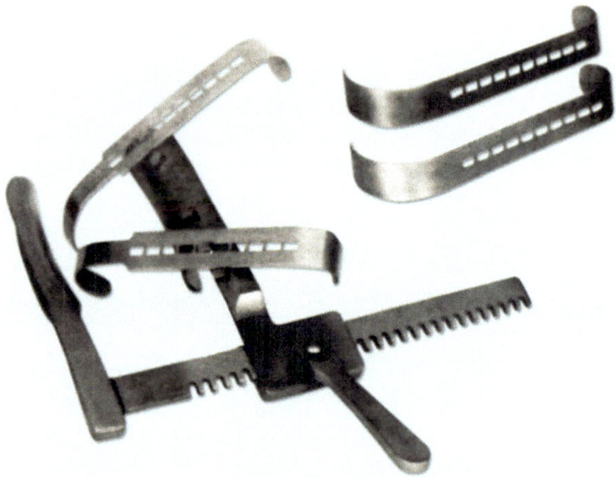

Fig. 3.20: Carpentier retractor

- Especially designed retractor for mitral valve surgery
- Sternal blade has elevated hook like projection for fixing mitral retractors.

How to Use

- After sternotomy, instrument should be placed in such a way that pinion-rack comes towards leg end
- After opening left atrium adequate size mitral retractor placed and fixed to sternal slot followed by other retractor as shown in Figure 3.20.

Advantage

- Good exposure of mitral valve so ideal for mitral valve repair surgery
- Same exposure throughout procedure
- No extra-assistance required to hold retractor.

Cosgrove Retractor

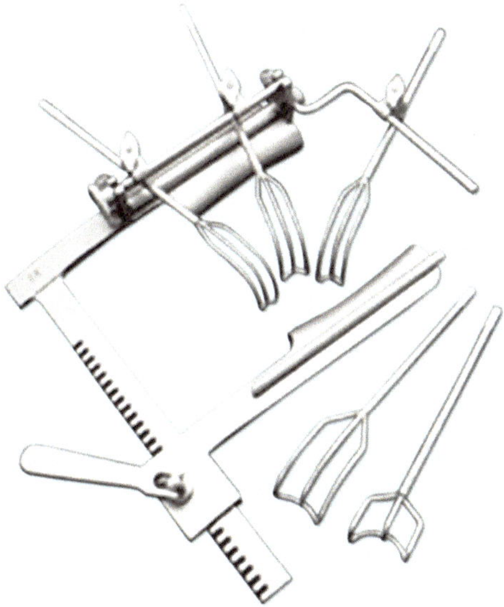

Fig. 3.21: Cosgrove retractor

- This is a selfretaining mitral valve retractor
- Sternal retractor has been modified for attachment of mitral valve retractor or valve retractors (Fig. 3.21).

Advantage

- Better exposure of mitral valve
- No assistance required
- Retraction can be done laterally also as there is a lateral extension road where instrument can be fixed (Fig. 3.22).

IMA Retractor

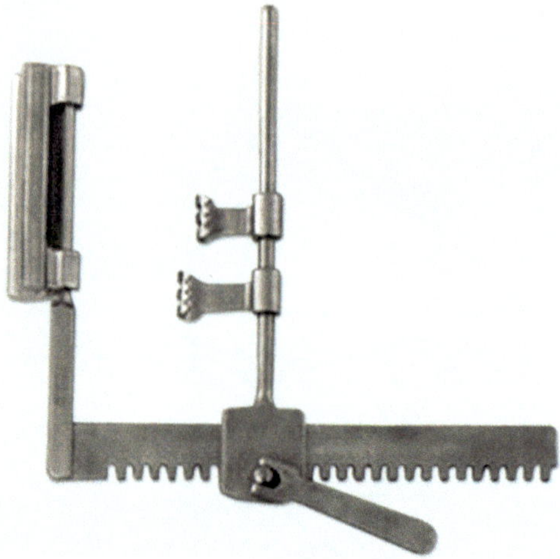

Fig. 3.22: Cosgrove's ready to use

- This instrument gives good exposure of internal mammary artery as it lifts up the sternum
- Retractor has supporting blade on one side while 2 mobile hooks on other side.

Method of Use

- After sternotomy, place supporting blade on right side of sternum, place both hook below left part of sternum
- Gently support rack from back side and open the retractor, as it opens, right side of sternum goes down while left side lifts up
- Care should be taken that resting blade should not compress cardiac chamber.

Rib Retractors

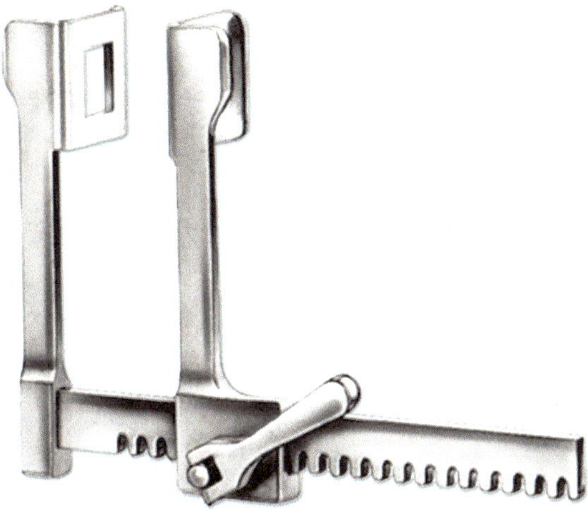

Fig. 3.23: Finochietto rib retractor

Finochietto Rib retractors

- Rack and pinion action (Fig. 3.23)
- Different sizes of blades are available.

Uses

In thoracotomy procedure to retract the rib like PDA ligation, coarctation repair, BT shunt.

- Posterolateral thoracotomy for ASD closure and mitral valve surgeries
- Used in ministernotomy for sternal retractors.

Modification

- Burford-Finochietto rib retractors
- This instrument has detachable blades (Fig. 3.24).

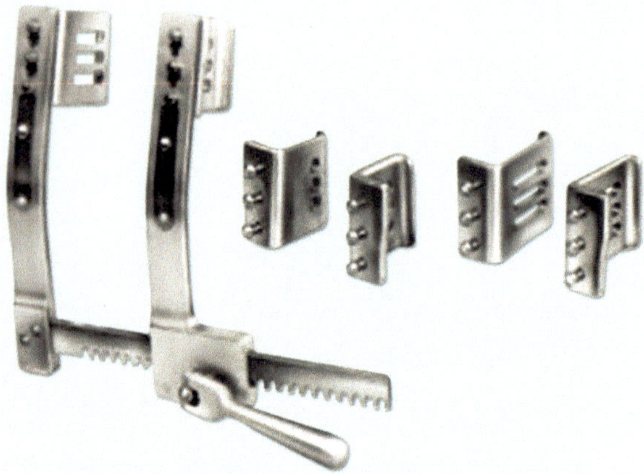

Fig. 3.24: Burford–Finochietto rib retractor

Tuffier Rib Retractor

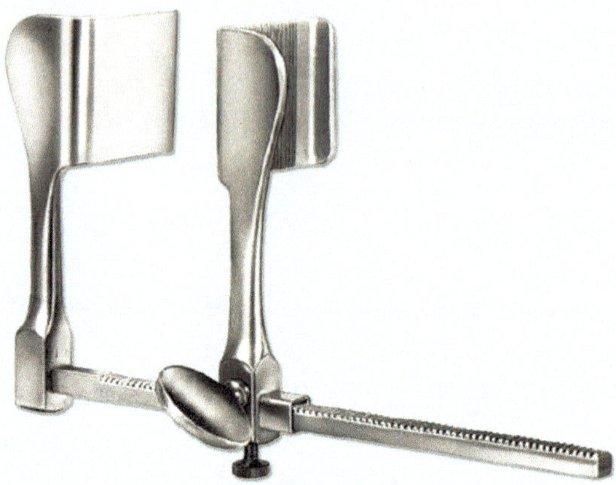

Fig. 3.25: Tuffier rib retractor

- Ratchet action
- Blade without hole
- Blade has serrations for grip (Fig. 3.25).

REFERENCES

1. Bonfils-Roberts EA. The rib spreader: a chapter in the history of thoracic surgery. Chest. 1972;61:469-74.
2. Deysine M and Uriburu JV. Enrique and Ricardo Finochietto: surgery, the ultimate devotion. Surgery. 1973;73:490-9.
3. Varea E. Enrique Finochietto (1881-1948) invest Urol. 1979;16:307-8.

CHAPTER

4

Forceps

HISTORY

Howard A Kelly (1858–1943)

First professor of gynecology and obstetrics at John Hopkins, Howard A Kelly (Fig. 4.1) assisted in fostering many surgical techniques and procedures involving the female reproductive and genitourinary tract. Kelly clamp is one of the most widely used and known surgical instrument.[1,2]

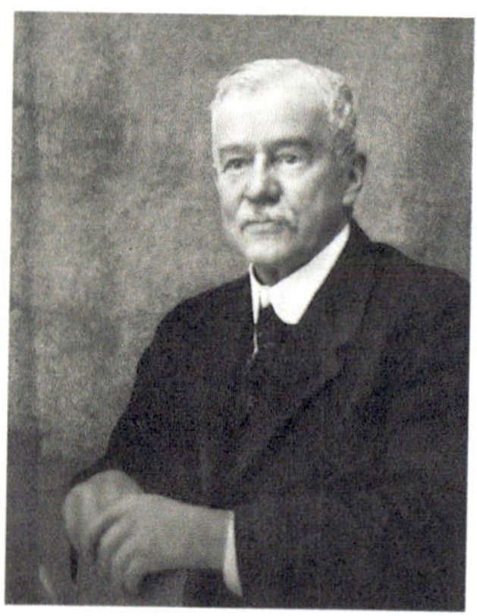

Fig. 4.1: Howard A Kelly

William Wayne Babcock (1872-1963)

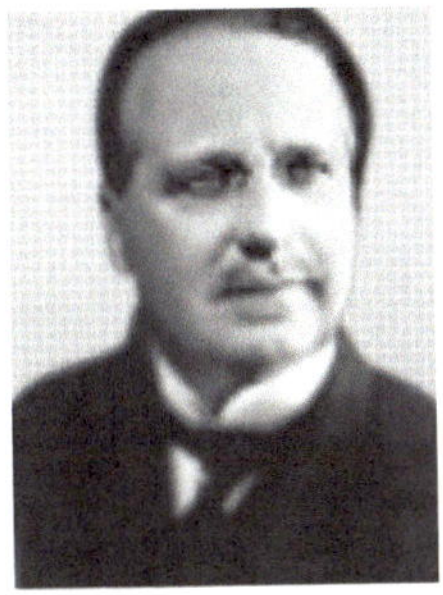

Fig. 4.2: William Wayne Babcock

William Wayne Babcock (Fig. 4.2) was recognized for his contribution in the field of colon and rectal surgery. He developed clamp which is widely used in many surgical specialties.[3]

- In any surgery forceps are used mainly to hold tissue for traction or apposition
- Ideal tissue forceps depends upon the tissue it has to handle
- It should have good grip with minimal tissue trauma
- Length of the forceps depends upon the depth of the area of surgery
- Forceps can be spring action type or lock type with 3 or more ratchets (catch, clamp and crush).

FORCEPS TYPES

Different forceps are described below.

Spencer Wells Hemostatic Forceps

They are curved and straight, transverse serrations, and are available in different sizes (Fig. 4.3).

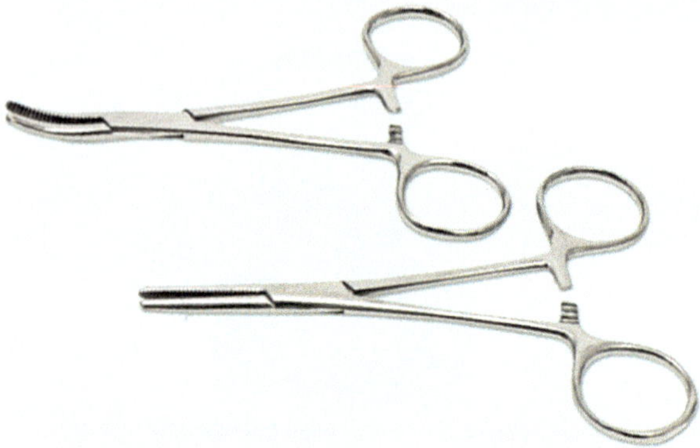

Fig. 4.3: Spencer wells hemostatic forceps

Uses in Cardiac Surgery

- To catch the bleeder
- To hold pericardial margin
- Holding other end of suture material (For this purpose tip has to be covered with soft rubber).
- Used as a blunt dissector

Kocher's Hemostatic Forceps

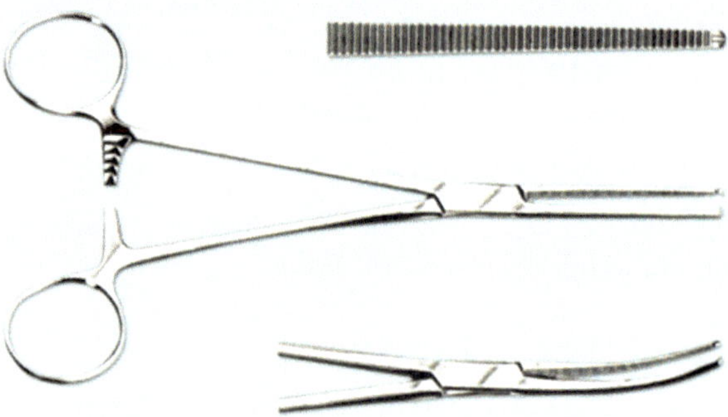

Fig. 4.4: Kocher's hemostatic forceps

- This has longer blades than artery forceps with teeth at the tip which helps holding tough tissue (Fig. 4.4)
- Curved and straight type.

Uses in Cardiac Surgery

- Leaflet holding in mitral valve replacement
- In constrictive pericarditis, it helps holding pericardium
- Holding steel wire ends during sternotomy closure.

Allis Tissue Forceps

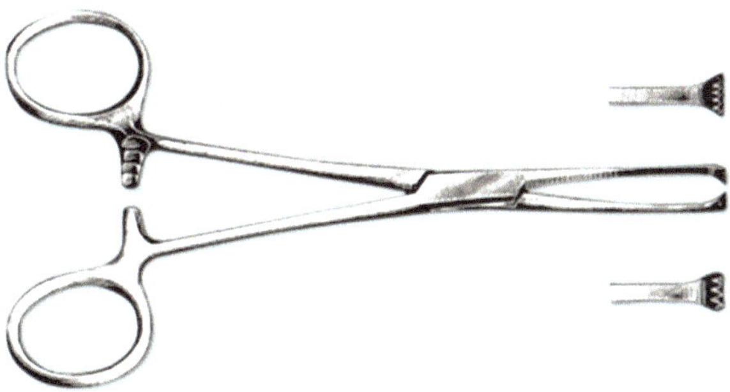

Fig. 4.5: Allis tissue forceps

- This instrument has straight blades which are slightly curved with the tip having interlocking teeth (Fig. 4.5).

Uses in Cardiac Surgery

- Holding pericardial edge
- Holding leaflet in mitral valve replacement.

Kelly Forceps

- Longer 8" Instrument with straight or curved blade
- Transverse serration in the blade (Fig. 4.6).

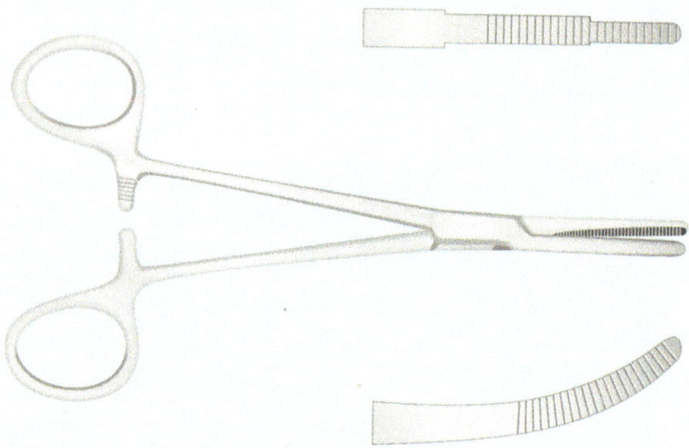

Fig. 4.6: Kelly forceps

Use in Cardiac Surgery

- Placing intercostal drainage tube
- Passing tube through incision for mediastinal tube
- Same like artery forceps.

Mixter

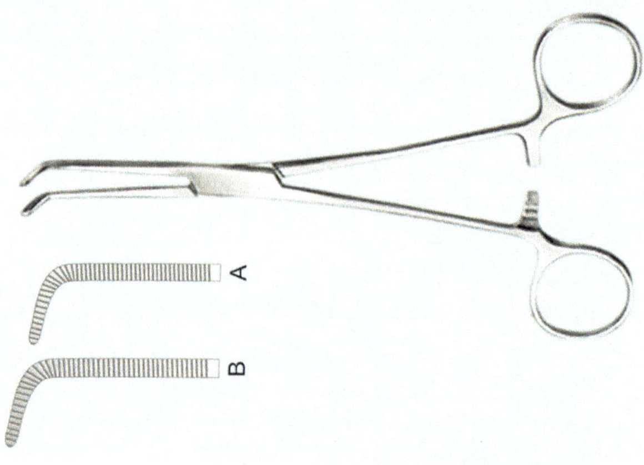

Fig. 4.7: Mixter

- Right angle curved blade with transverse serrations (Fig. 4.7)
- Different length available with tip blunt to sharp.

Uses

- Encircling of any vascular structure is useful
- SVC, IVC, Aorta, femoral artery, femoral vein, vertical vein, and PDA encircling
- Tying thymus after dividing into middle
- Stabilizing aorta during aortic cannulation
- Testing mechanical value disc movement after valve replacement surgery
- Retracting subvalvular apparatus during mitral valve repair.

Care During Use

- During encircling vascular structure movement of mixture should be gentle and it should be circular not perpendicular to vessel, to avoid injury to posterior wall of vessel.

Gerald Forceps

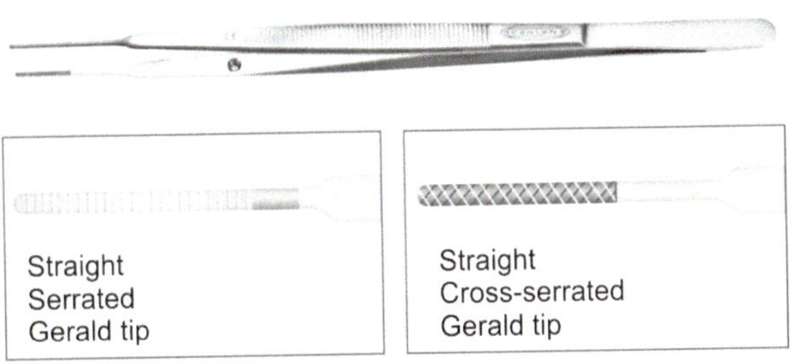

Fig. 4.8: Gerald forceps

- This is a forceps with finer tip having transverse serrations. Serrated finer grip (Fig. 4.8)

- Tip of the forceps can be tooth , nontooth or cross serrated also. Diffrent sizes are available.

Use

- During intracardiac suturing like ASD closure, VSD closure, TOF repair it is used for sutures 5/0 or 6/0
- Dissection of MAPCA, PDA, Pulmonary artery
- Proximal anastomosis of graft in CABG.

Duval Forceps

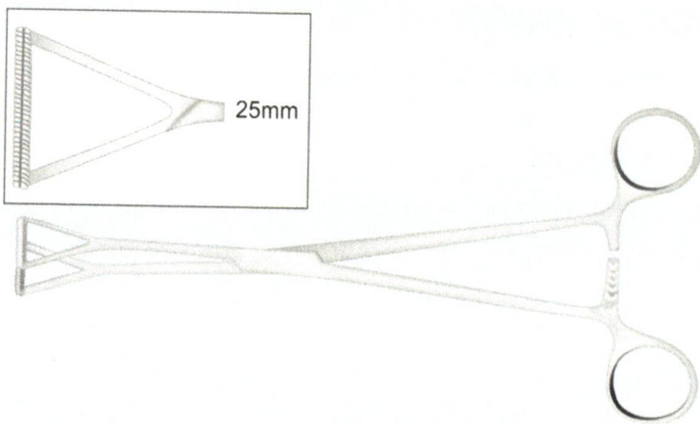

Fig. 4.9: Duval forceps

- Long blade with triangle at end (Fig. 4.9)
- Transverse serration.

Use

- Lung tissue holding during various procedure on lung, like decortication, pneumonectomy, lobectomy.

Rumel

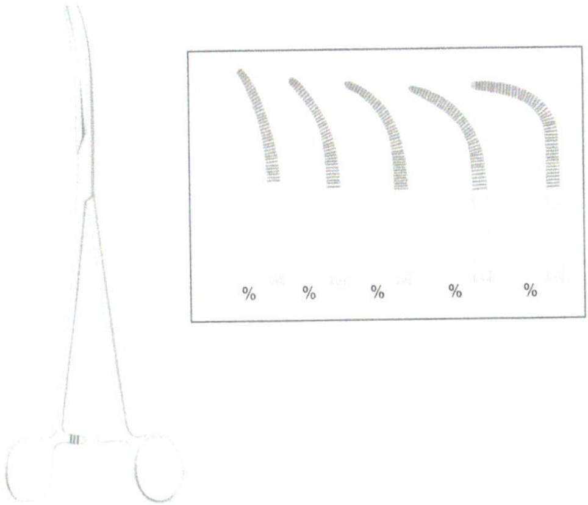

Fig. 4.10: Rumel

- It has long length of blade with transverse serrations. Different angulation blades are available. Blades are partially serrated and partially smooth (Fig. 4.10).

Use

Same like Kelly's forceps.

Russian Forceps

- This is a spring action forceps with round hole tip at end
- Toothed serration at tip of forceps (Fig. 4.11).

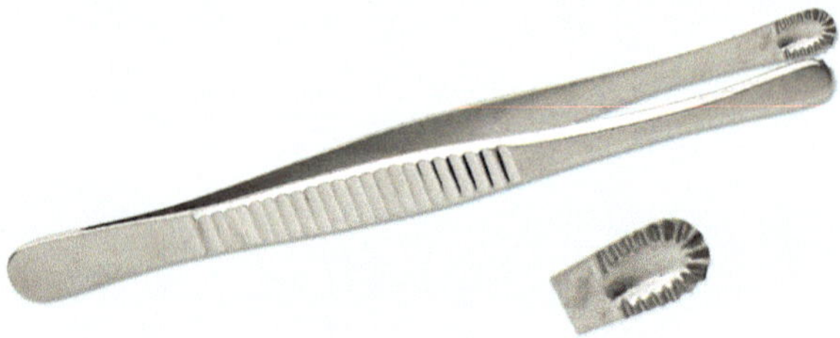

Fig. 4.11: Russian forceps

Use

- Removal of clot from LA or LV cavity
- During re-exploration cleaning pericardial cavity
- Holding pericardium in constrictive pericarditis
- Decortication of lung.

Vascular Forceps

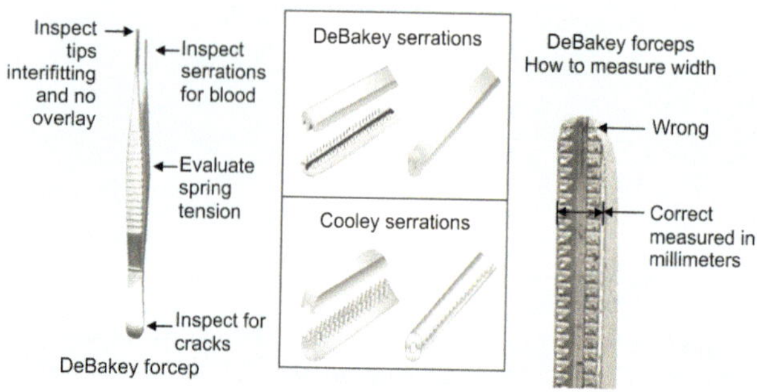

Fig. 4.12: Types of serration

- Different types of vascular forceps available with different patterns of serrations (Fig. 4.12)
- They are named according to pattern of serrations.

Fine Serration

- Castaneda type
- Single row of fine serrations which are precisely meshed (Fig. 4.13)

Fig. 4.13: Fine serration

Use

Handling of small vessels.

Cooley's Type Serrations

- 2 × 2 vascular teeth
- In this type double row of finely serrated teeth arranged in opposing row.

Advantage

- Better grip of vessels
- Less tissue injury.

DeBakey Type Serrations

- 1 × 2 vascular teeth
- DeBakey type has two rows of finely serrated teeth on one blade and one row on the opposing blade.

Advantage

- Triangular, good grip
- Better approximation of tissue with less tissue injury.

DeBakey Forceps

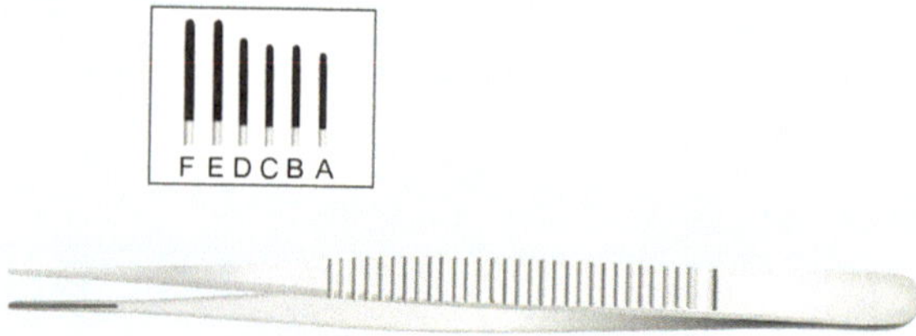

Fig. 4.14: DeBakey forceps

- Different length available
- Different jaw size available
- 1 mm for finer works on coronary arteries (Fig. 4.14)
- 2–3 mm for relatively bigger vessels.

CASTANEDA VASCULAR FORCEPS

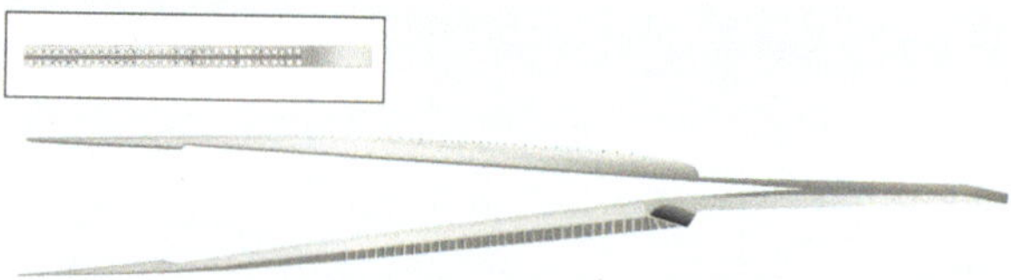

Fig. 4.15: Castaneda vascular forceps

- Fine serrated teeth jaw
- Different jaw and length sizes available (Fig. 4.15).

Cooley's Vascular Tissue Forceps

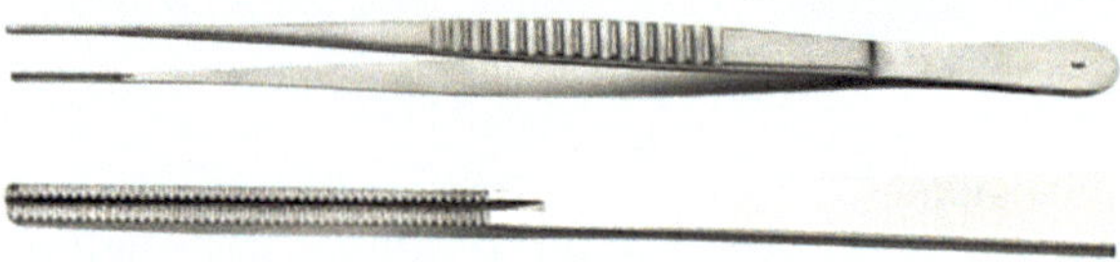

Fig. 4.16: Cooley's vascular tissue forceps

- 2 × 2 Serrated jaw
- Different length and jaw sizes available (Fig. 4.16).

Ring Tip Vascular Forceps

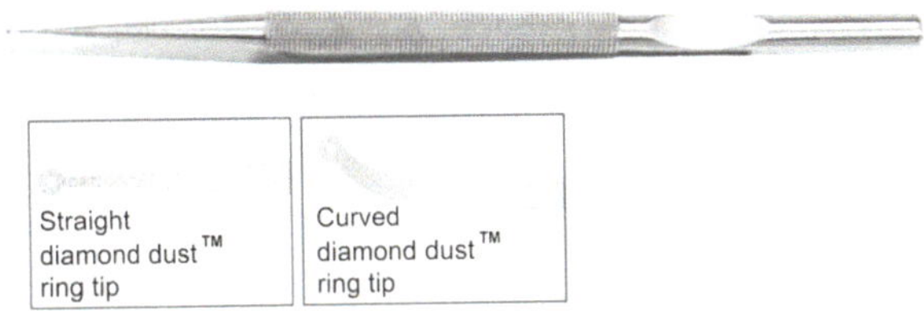

Fig. 4.17: Ring tip vascular forceps

- This is a vascular forceps without serration with round-shaped tip (Fig. 4.17).

Use

- IMA preparation
- Anastomosis of IMA to LAD or diagonal vessel
- Whenever 8/0 prolene to be used for suturing, this forceps is useful.

Angle Vascular Forceps (IMA Forceps)

- Vascular forceps with curved blade with DeBakey type serration.
- Different angulation 90, 120, 140, available (Fig. 4.18).

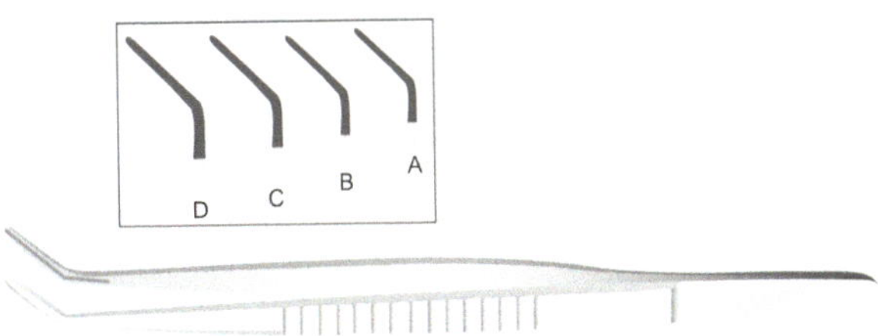

Fig. 4.18: IMA forceps

Use

- IMA dissection
- Hemostasis below sternum
- MAPCA dissection in TOF, pulmonary atresia.

Daicoff Vascular and Needle Pulling Forceps

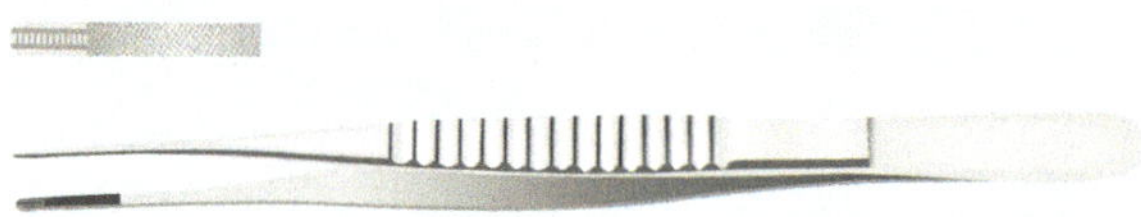

Fig. 4.19: Daicoff vascular and needle pulling forceps

- Jaw of this forceps has combination of cooley's serration at tips, finner criss-cross serration in rest of the area.

Uses

- Vascular forceps
- Needle pulling forceps.

Foss Tube milking Forceps

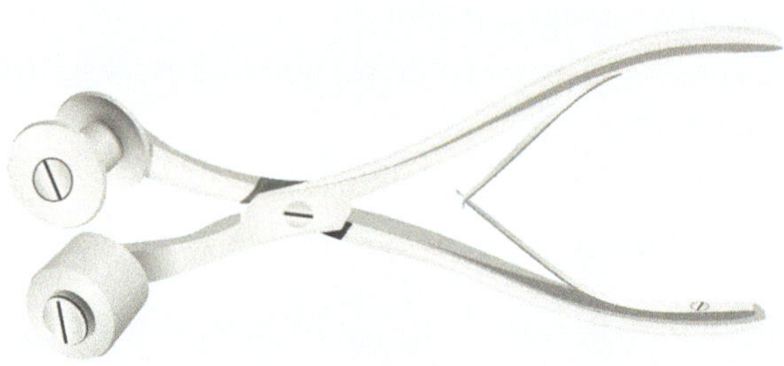

Fig. 4.20: Foss tube milking forceps

- This instrument has good grip with spring action at one end while other end has 2 cylindrical rotatable cuff (Fig. 4.20).

Uses

- Milking the tube for prevention of tube block by blood clot.

Method

- Apply paraffin over chest drain, hold tube proximally with one hand while with the other hand hold tube with the instrument and slide out and release it.

REFERENCES

1. Allen PM and Setze TK. Howard Atwood Kelly 91858-1943). South Med J. 1991;84:361-8.
2. Logon LD and Howard A Kelly's development as an academician: some insight from his letters to Robert P Harris. Trans Stud Coll Physicians Phila. 2002;24:93-136.
3. Corman ML. William Wayne Babcock 1872-1963. Dis Colon Rectum. 1991;32:442-7.

CHAPTER

5

Scissors

HISTORY

Willis Potts (1895-1968)

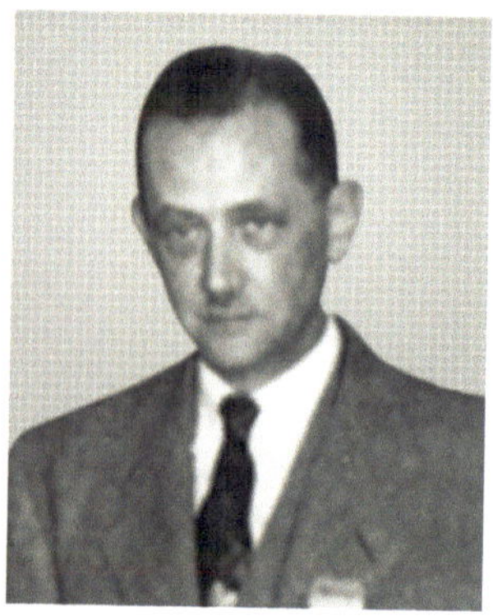

Fig. 5.1: Wills Potts

Willis Potts (Fig. 5.1) developed the palliative procedure to treat TOF: Potts shunt anastomosis between descending aorta and left pulmonary artery.

He developed fine scissors and forceps, which are still used today.[1]

William J Mayo and Charles H Mayo

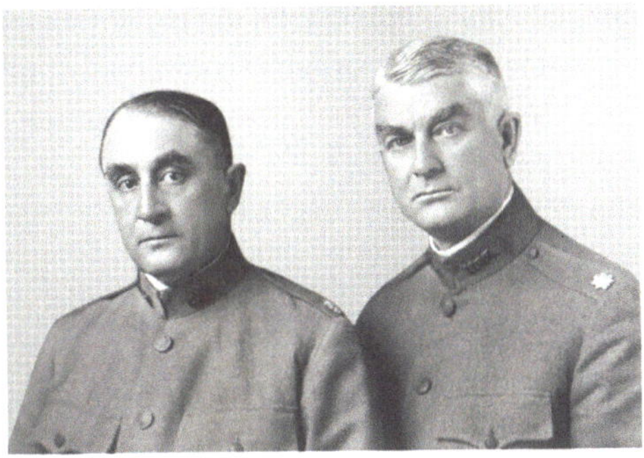

Fig. 5.2: William J Mayo and Charles H Mayo

They developed Mayo scissors at Mayo Clinic Rochester, MN.[2]

Dr Myron Metzenbaum

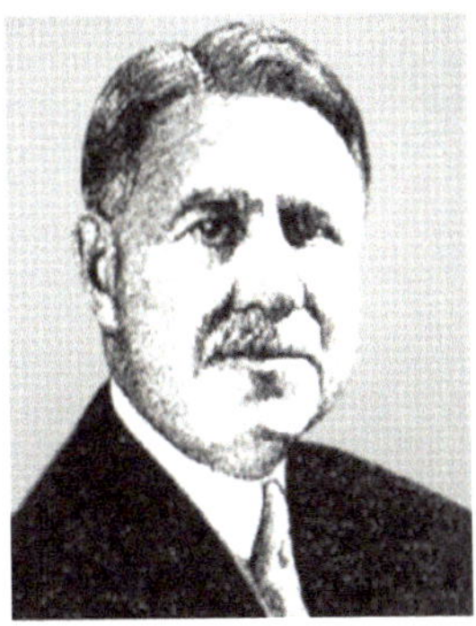

Fig. 5.3: Dr Myron Metzenbaum

An otolaryngologist, Dr Myron Metzenbaum (Fig. 5.3) was a leader in the treatment of cleft lip and palate. He developed scissors that bears his name.[3]

- Scissors are used to cut tissue or vessels
- According to type of use different kind of scissors with different size, shape and blades are made
- Razor sharp cutting edge for gentle cutting with minimum force
- Wave cut blade—prevents tissue from slipping out during the cutting process
- Commonly used scissors in cardiac surgery are mentioned below.

DISSECTING TISSUE SCISSOR

Mayo Scissors

Identification

- Tough wider blades with sharp edge of blade
- Straight and curved types (Fig. 5.4).

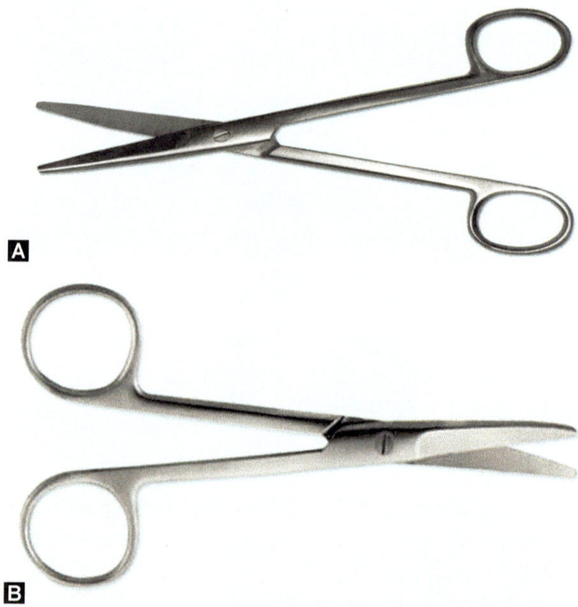

Fig. 5.4: Mayo Scissors

Uses

- As a sternal cutter in neonates and infant
- To cut pacing wire
- To cut tube during cardiopulmonary bypass
- Pericardial patch harvest
- Pericardial adhesions separation in redo sternotomy
- To cut sutures.

Metzenbaum Scissor

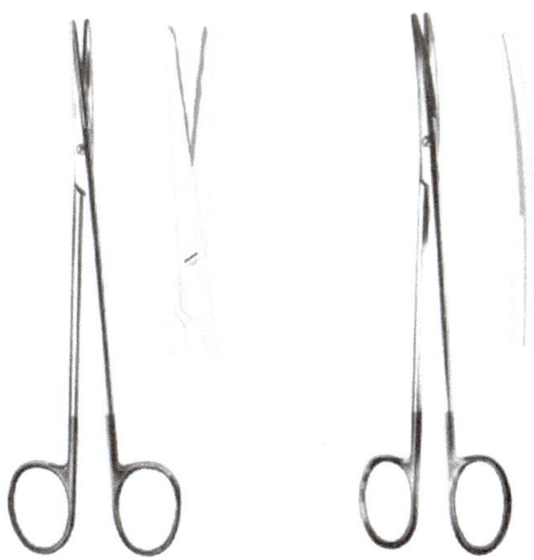

Fig. 5.5: Metzenbaum scissor

Identification

- Long thin blades with sharp or serrated edge
- Straight and curved types (Fig. 5.5).

Uses

- Pericardiotomy
- Pericardial dissection

- Opening of right atrium, or left atrium.
- Aortotomy in aortic valve replacement.

SCISSORS VASCULAR

Diethrich Valve Scissor

Identification

- Long thin blade with serration
- Curved anteriorly.

Uses

- Mitral valve leaflet cutting
- Aortic valve leaflet.

Litwak Mitral Valve Scissor

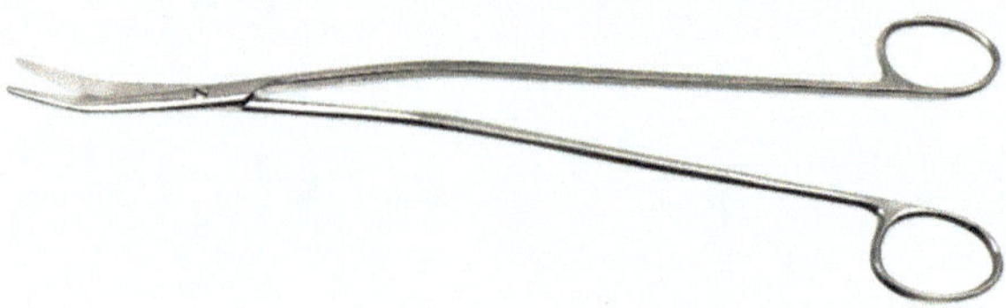

Fig. 5.6: Litwak mitral valve scissor

- Angled on side and curved blade (Fig. 5.6).

Potts–Smith Vascular Scissors

Identification (Fig. 5.7)

- Short blade with pointed sharp tip
- Angulated by side from joint
- 25°, 45° and 60°, 90°, 125° angle available
- Spring action [Yasargil modification available].

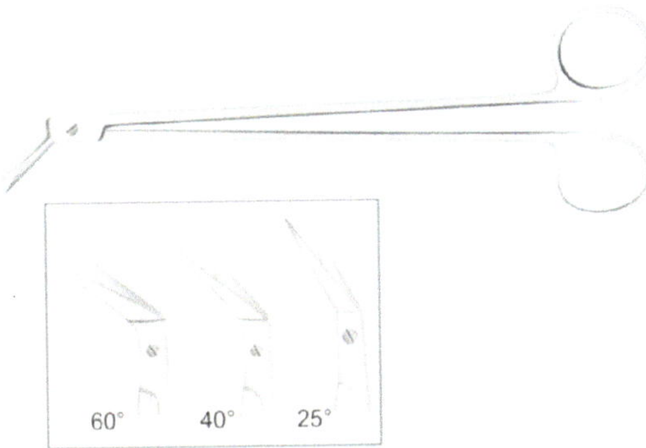

Fig. 5.7: Potts–Smith vascular scissors

Uses

- Arteriotomy enlargement
- Venotomy enlargement
- Finer dissection in neonatal cardiac surgery
- Excision of coronary artery button in arterial switch procedure, Ross procedure.

DeBakey Vascular Scissors

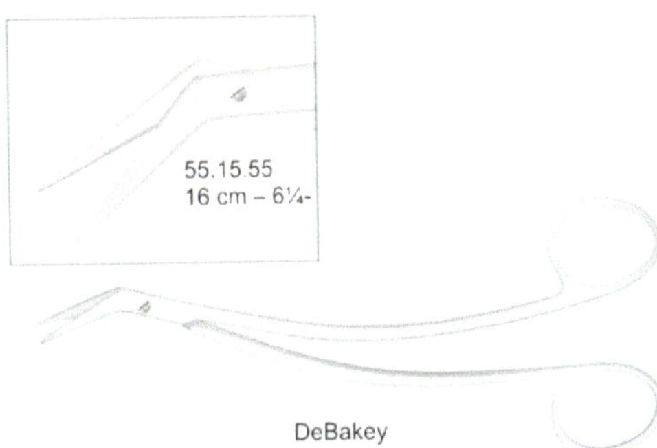

Fig. 5.8: DeBakey

Uses

- Same as potts-smith vascular scissor (Fig. 5.8).

Tenotomy Scissors

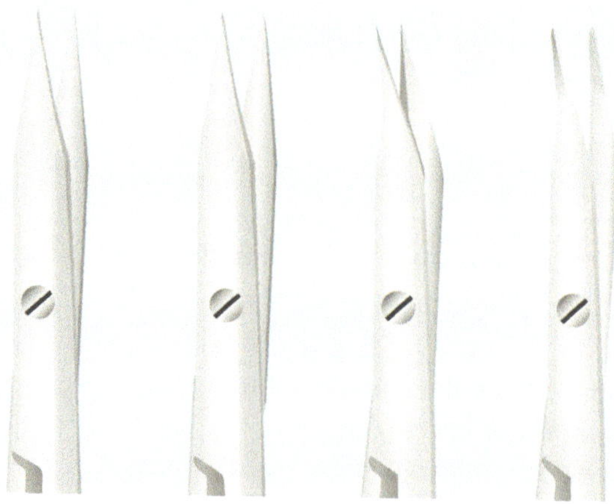

Fig. 5.9: Tenotomy scissors

Identification (Fig. 5.9)

- Tip is tapered and pointed like dolphin fin
- Potts type and Metzenbaum type are available.

Uses

- Finer intracardiac excision and resection.

CORONARY ARTERY SCISSORS

Diethrich Coronary Artery Scissor

- Fine tip, small curved blade
- 25°, 45°, 60°, 90°, angle available (Fig. 5.10).

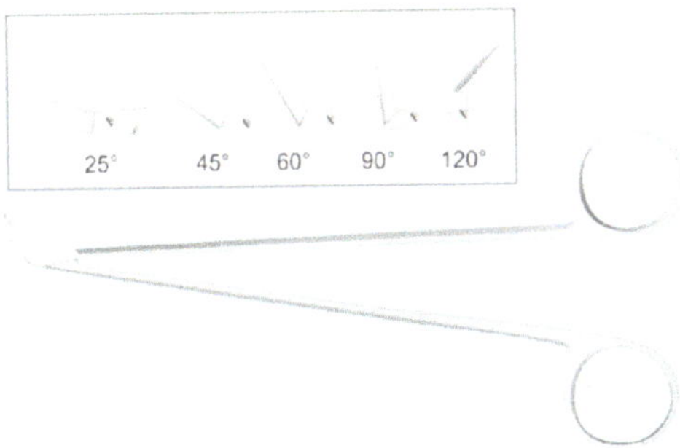

Fig. 5.10: Diethrich coronary artery scissor

Uses

- Coronary arteriotomy.

Diethrich Circumflex Artery Scissor

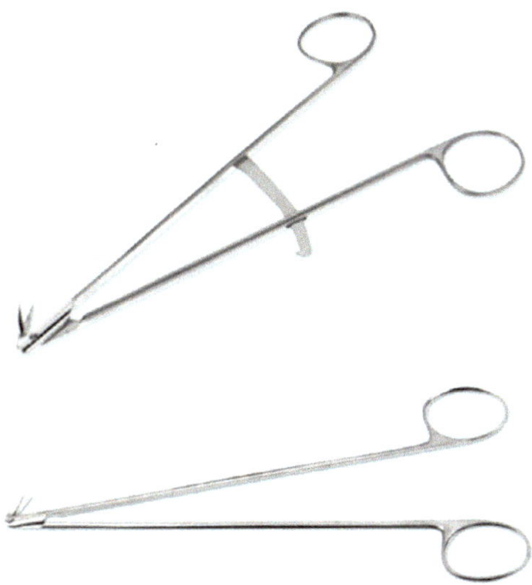

Fig. 5.11: Diethrich circumflex artery scissor

- Fine tip, small, 125º angled curved blade
- Stabilizing bar at middle of the shaft (Fig. 5.11).

Uses

- Arteriotomy for OM, OM2 modification. LAWRIE circumflex scissor.
- Without stabilizing middle shaft.

Favaloro Coronary Scissors

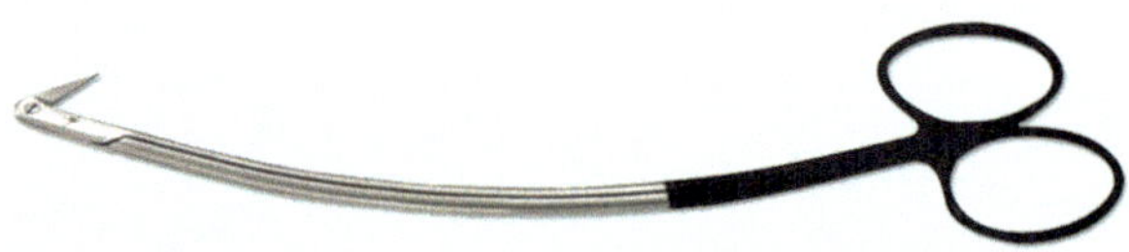

Fig. 5.12: Favaloro coronary scissors

- Fine tip short blade angled at 130º.
- Shank is curved (Fig. 5.12).

Jones IMA Scissors

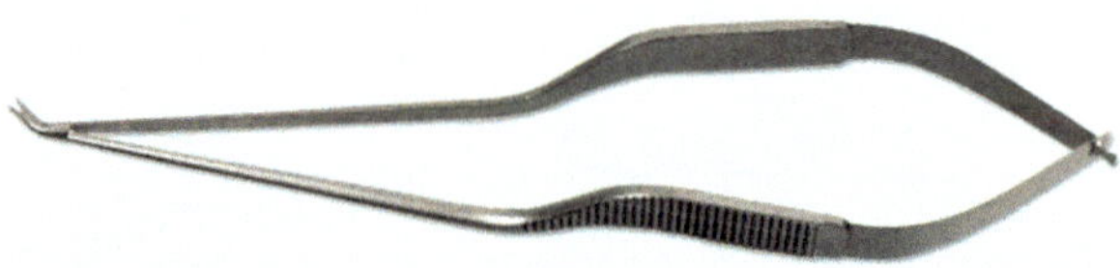

Fig. 5.13: Jones IMA scissors

- Flat handle spring action, curved body (Fig. 5.13)
- Blade very thin, short and pointed with different angle.

Use

- IMA preparation and arteriotomy.

REFERENCES

1. Baffes TG, Potts WJ: Ann Thor Surg. 1987;44:92-6.
2. Nelson CW. The surgical careers of the Mayo Brothers. Mayo Clinic. 1998;73:716.
3. Metson R, Myron F (Metzenbaum, MD) Otolaryngol HeadNeck Surg.1994:110:477-81.

CHAPTER

6

Needle Holder

HISTORY

Ramon Castroviejo (1904–1987)

The son of a prominent Spanish ophthalmologist, Ramon Castroviejo (Fig. 6.1) became a pioneer in advancing the field of eye surgery. He developed numerous fine surgical tools, including the needle driver.[1]

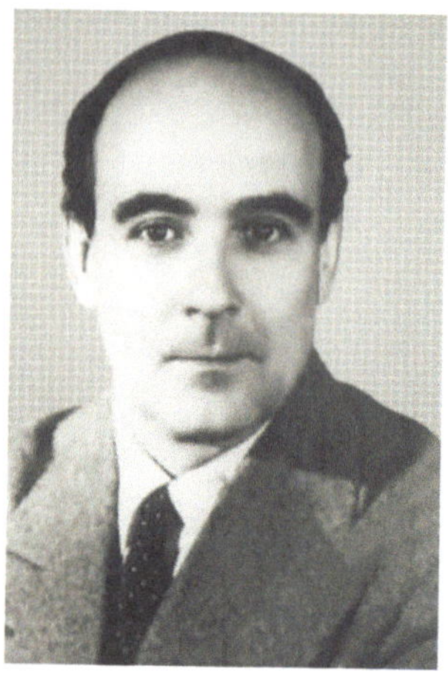

Fig. 6.1: Ramon Castroviejo

NEEDLE HOLDER

- Different types of needle holders are used in cardiac surgery depending upon the type of needle to be used.
- Needle holder tip plays major roles in quality which are mentioned below.

TUNGSTEN CARBIDE TIP

- It is approximately two times stiffer than steel
- Tungsten carbide tip with fine serration provides tough grip to needle and it last longer (Fig. 6.2).

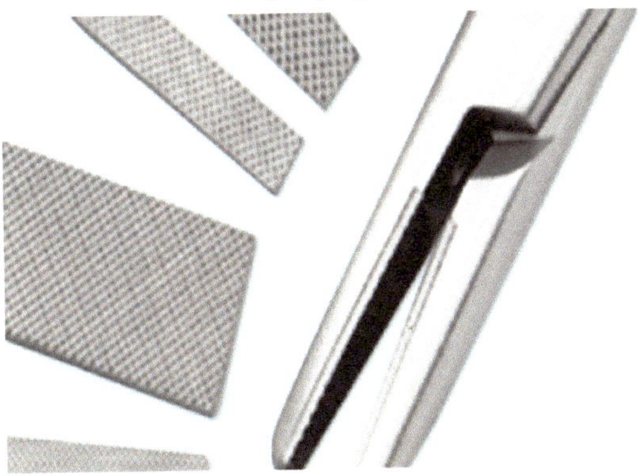

Fig. 6.2: Tungsten carbide tip

Diamond Dust Coated Tip

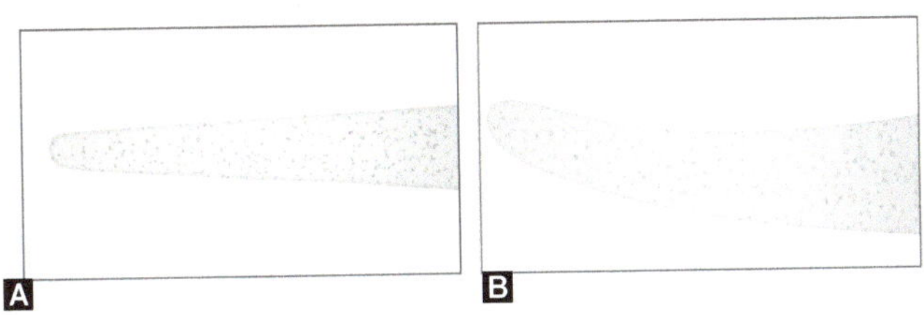

Figs 6.3A and B: (A) Straight diamond dust™ jaws; (B) Curved diamond dust™ jaws

- Diamond dust is leftover material from cutting diamonds and is extremely hard.
- It is coated on tip of finer needle holders which gives strength to the tip and good grip to smaller needles like 6/0, 7/0, 8/0 during suturing (Fig. 6.3).

Standard Serrated Tip

- Tip of needle holder has been serrated for good grip of needle
- Serration can be transverse, fine or criss-cross.

Mayo–Hegar Needle Holder

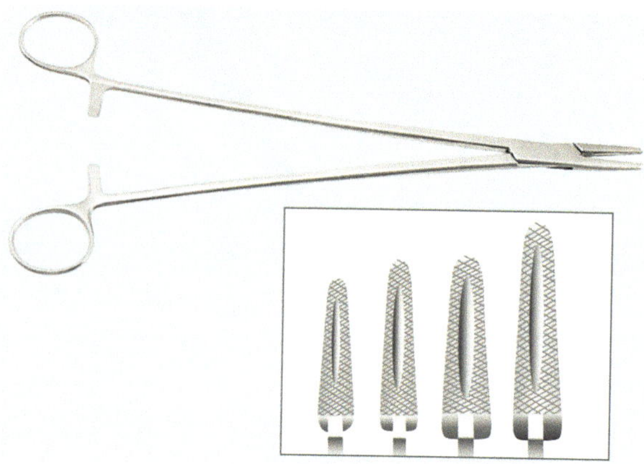

Figs 6.4: Mayo–Hegar needle holder

Identification: Heavy tip with groove in middle (Fig. 6.4).

Uses

- Handling 1/0 , 2/0 sutures.
- As a sternal wire bending purpose.

Crilewood Needle Holder

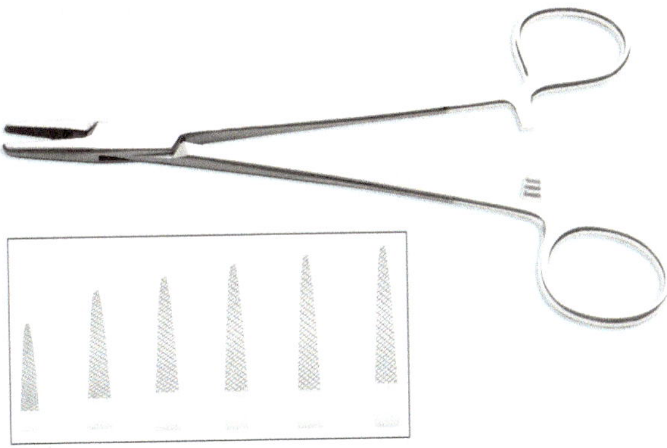

Figs 6.5: Crilewood needle holder

Specification

- Finer jaw than Mayo-Hegar needle holder.
- Tip serrations various, mostly medium type serrations (Fig. 6.5).

Uses

- For 3/0 and 4/0 sutures.

DeBakey Needle Holder

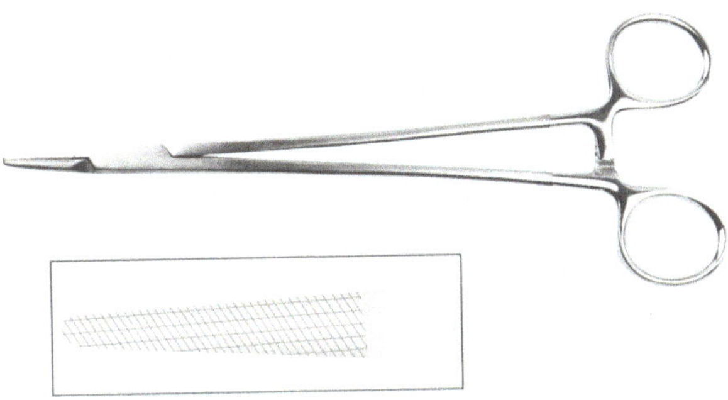

Fig. 6.6: DeBakey needle holder

Specification

- This needle holder tip is finer than Crile wood with finer serrations.

Uses

- For 4/0 and 5/0 suture this can be used.

Ryder

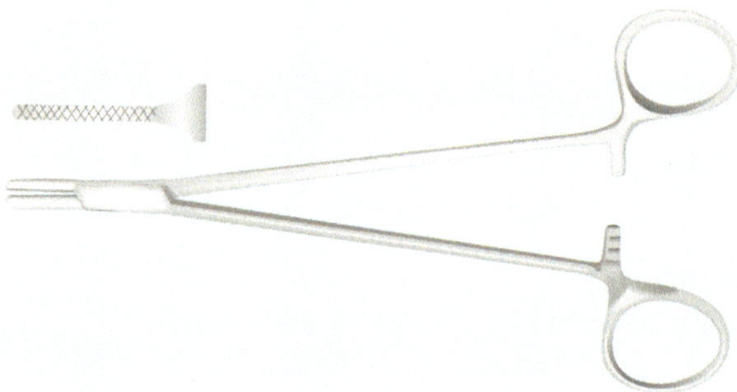

Fig. 6.7: Ryder

Specification

- Tip of the jaw is tapered like dolphin jaw
- Finer serrations tip can be tungsten or diamond dust coated (Fig. 6.7).

Uses

- For 5/0 and 6/0 sutures this can be used.

Sarot Needle Holder

Identification

- Handle is curved
- Jaw small with fine tip and finer serrations (Fig. 6.8).

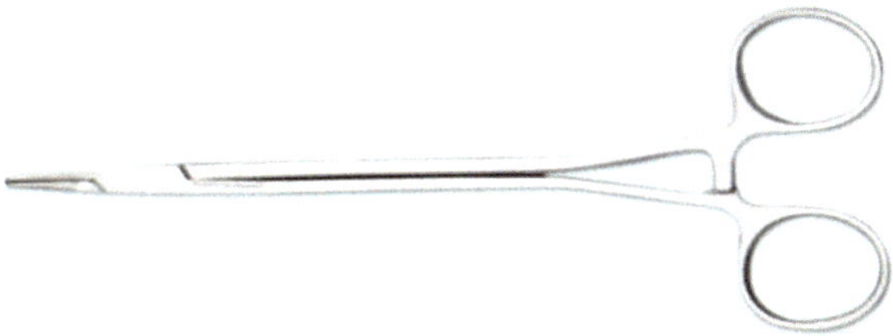

Fig. 6.8: Sarot needle holder

Uses

- For sutures 5/0 and 6/0 this needle holder can be used.

Castroviejo Needle Holder

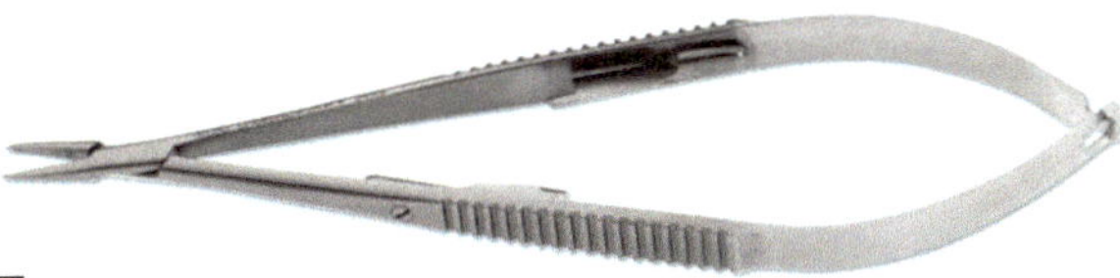

A

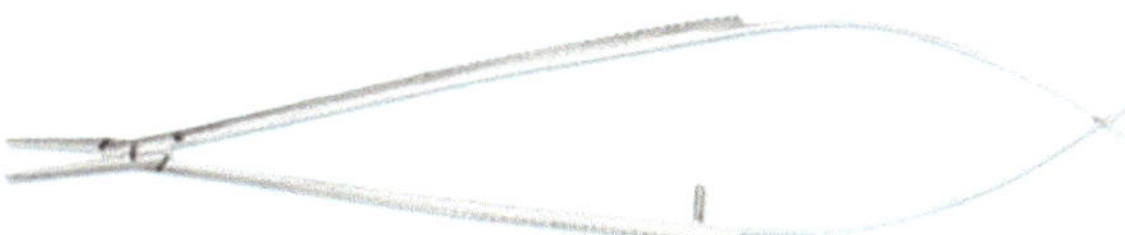

B

Figs 6.9A and B: Castroviejo needle holder

Identification

- Jaw is small with fine tip
- Spring action with or without locking mechanism
- Handle is either flat or round shaped
- Tip may be standard or diamond dust coated
- Titanium also available which is lighter in weight
- Angled tip is available for suturing in depth with difficult angle (Fig. 6.9).

Uses

- This needle holder is easy to maneuver so it is widely used for intracardiac suturing.
- Sutures like 6/0, 7/0, 8/0 needles are mainly used.
- Widely used in coronary artery anastomosis.

Sternal Needle Holder

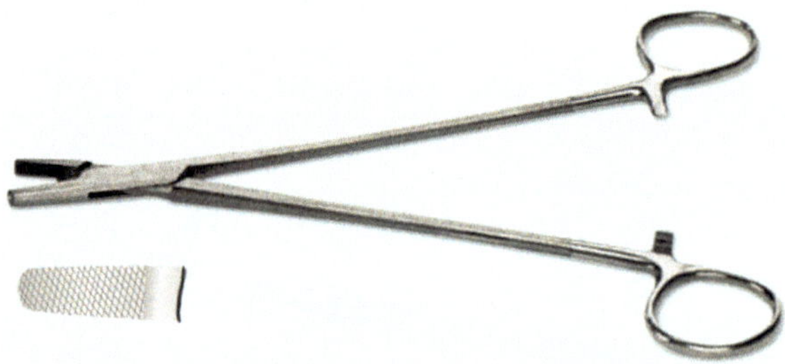

Fig. 6.10: Sternal needle holder

Identification

Jaw is larger and tough with tungsten carbide coated tip (Fig. 6.10).

Use

During sternum closure for 4 and 6 stainless steel wire holding.

REFERENCES

1. Murube J. Ramon Castroviejo centenary:a life dedicated to corneal transplantation. Surg opthalmol. 2005;50:215-25.

CHAPTER

7

Dilators and Dissectors

DILATORS

Garrett Vascular Dilators

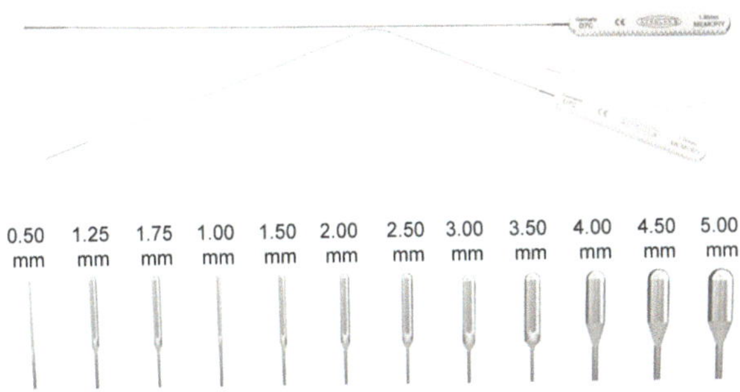

Fig. 7.1: Garrett vascular dilators—oval tip

- Oval tip with malleable shaft (Fig. 7.1).

Uses

- Sizing of vessel
- Probing of vessel to know patency
- To know course of vessel during cardioplegic, collapsed heart.

HEGAR DILATOR

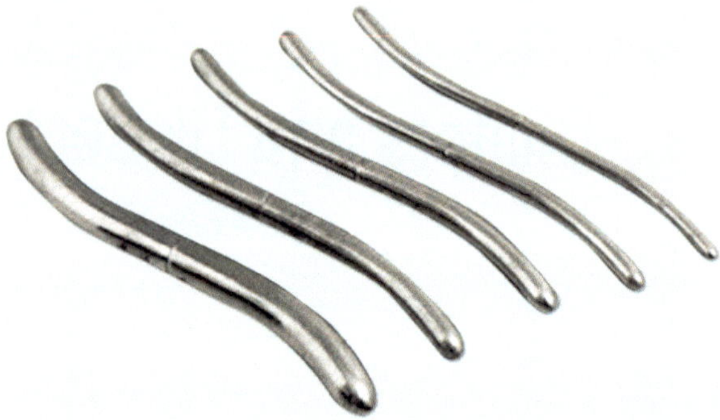

Fig. 7.2: Hegar dilators

Use

- Sizing of RVOT, LVOT (Fig. 7.2)
- Dilation of RVOT, LVOT, mitral valve.

Myocardial Dilator

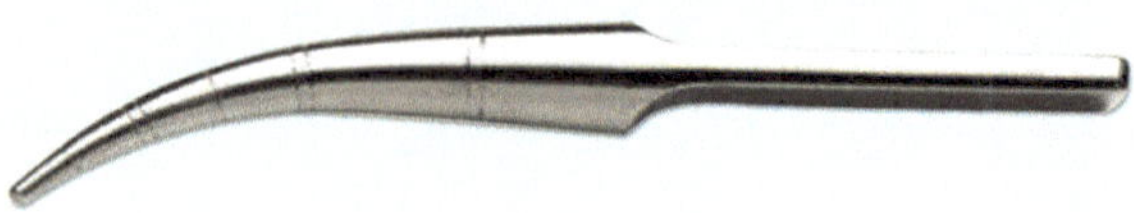

Fig. 7.3: Myocardial dilator

- 2 mm tip which graduates to 17.5 mm (Fig. 7.3)

TUBBS DILATOR

This dilator is transventricular type.

Originally, Logan and Turner made it followed by several modifications introduced by PK Sen, Cooley, Beck, Glenn, and finally, Tubb.

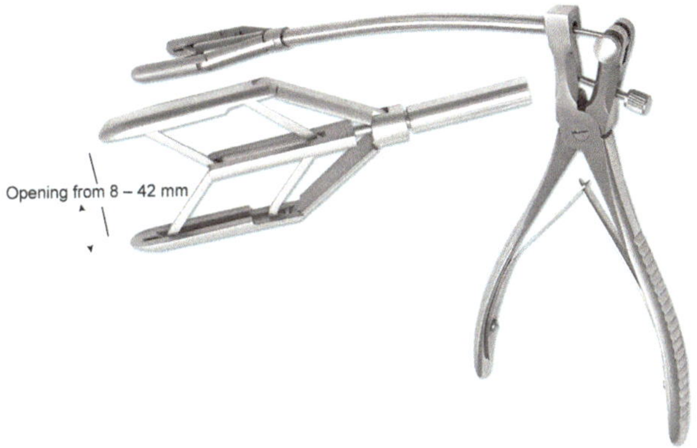

Fig. 7.4: Tubbs dilator

Tubb introduced a screw to enable a predetermine opening distance of the dilator (Fig. 7.4)

Q. How to check the dilator before Use?

- It should open smoothly
- Open against resistance
- Close completely
- Its blade should not rotate.

Q. What complications may occur during Close Mitral Commissurotomy?

- LV purse-string can cut through dilator stuck in open position
- Tip getting entangled
- Tearing of leaflet results in acute MR.

Q. In small LA how should you take purse-string?

At posterior aspect of LA extending over the pulmonary veins.

APPROXIMATORS (CONTRACTORS)

Bailey Rib Contractor

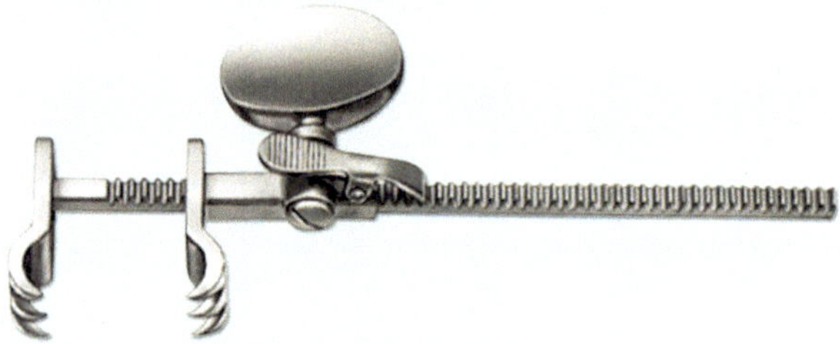

Fig. 7.5: Bailey rib contractors

- Ratchet action with curved pronged blade (Fig. 7.5).

Uses

- Rib approximation in thoracotomy closure time.

Lemmon Sternal Approximator

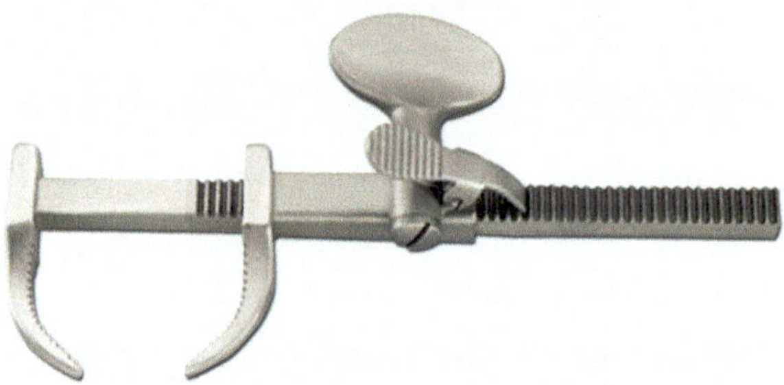

Fig. 7.6: Lemmon sternal approximator

Use

In sternal approximation (Fig. 7.6).

DISSECTORS

Duct Dissector

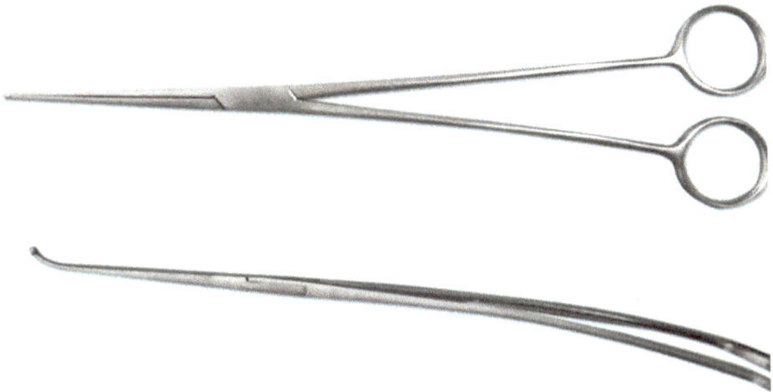

Fig. 7.7: Duct dissector

- Ball tip at end of blade
- No ratchets
- Straight, curved, and right angle tip available (Fig. 7.7).

Uses

- Dissection of PDA
- Dissection of pulmonary arteries and collaterals
- Useful in any blunt dissection.

Lemmon Intima Dissector

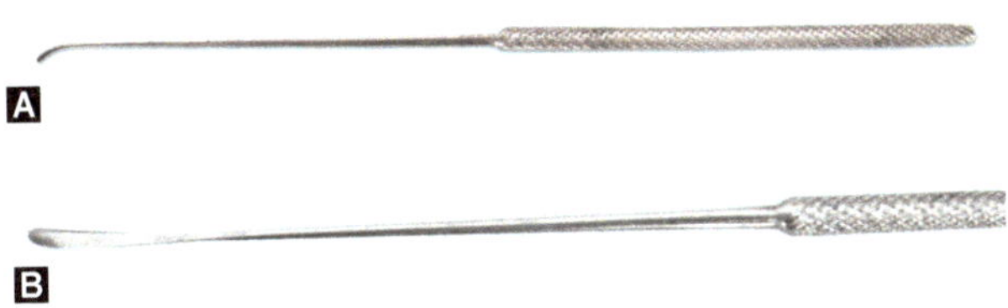

Figs 7.8A and B: Lemmon intima dissectors

Uses

- Endarterectomy
- Subaortic membrane resection
- Pilling of leaflet in rheumatic mitral valve disease (Fig. 7.8).

Rounger

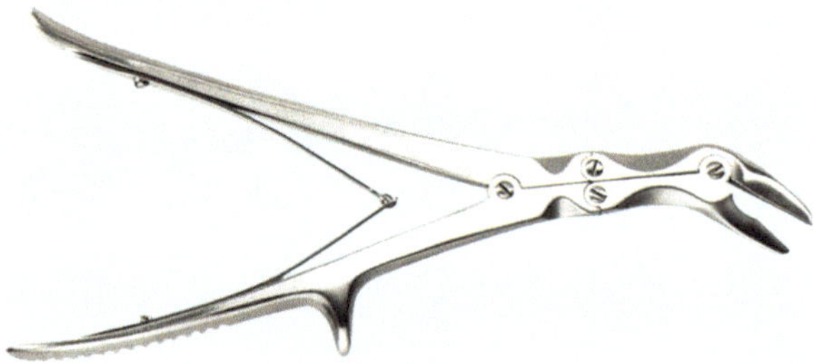

Fig. 7.9: Rounger

Uses

- It helps to remove calcium from calcified aortic valve and annulus.
- Annular debridement in infective endocarditis.

Different Types of Bone Roungers Available

Uses

Neebling of sternum in case of mediastinitis (Fig. 7.9).

CHAPTER

8

Suction Cannula

YANKAUER SUCTION TUBE

- Removable tip
- Tip has center as well as side holes
- Metal and plastic type available (Fig. 8.1).

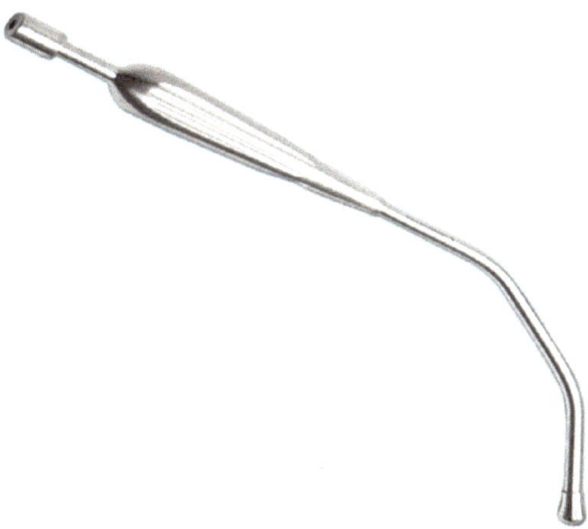

Fig. 8.1: Yankauer suction tube

Uses

- Suction of fluid or secretion in pericardial cavity

- After valve excision in aortic valve to remove calcium particle or small tissue piece from LV
- In re-exploration to clear pericardial cavity.

POOL SUCTION TUBE

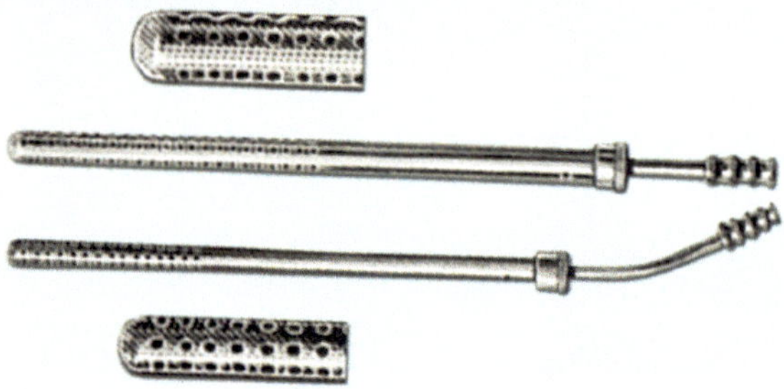

Fig. 8.2: Pool suction tubes

Identification

This suction has fenestrated tube over suction tube, so suction trauma can be minimized (Fig. 8.2).

Uses

Intracavitary suctioning to prevent damage to adjacent structure.

FRAZIER SUCTION TUBE

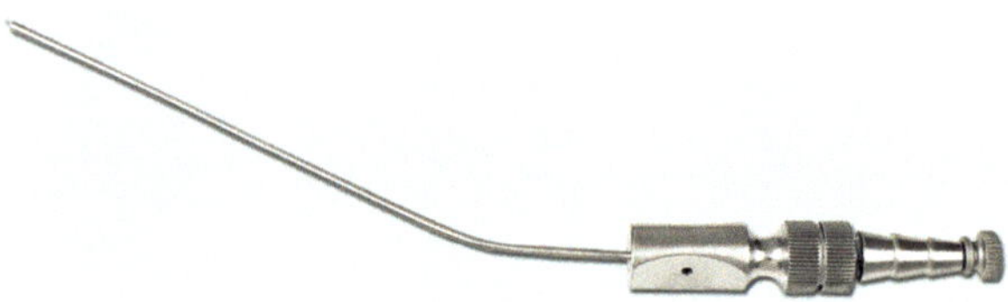

Fig. 8.3: Frazier suction tube

Angled thin tube suction with hole in handle to control suction power (Fig. 8.3).

Uses

- After arteriotomy, suction of blood during anastomosis
- Intracardiac repair in neonates and infants.

CARDIOTOMY SUCTION

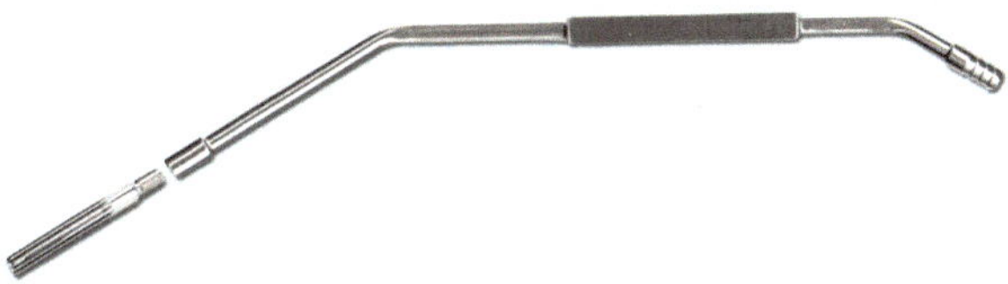

Fig. 8.4: Cardiotomy suction tip

Identification

- Longer multiple slot
- Tip can be removed for cleaning (Fig. 8.4).

Uses

- Suction of blood from pericardial cavity or cardiac cavity in open heart surgery.

BULLET

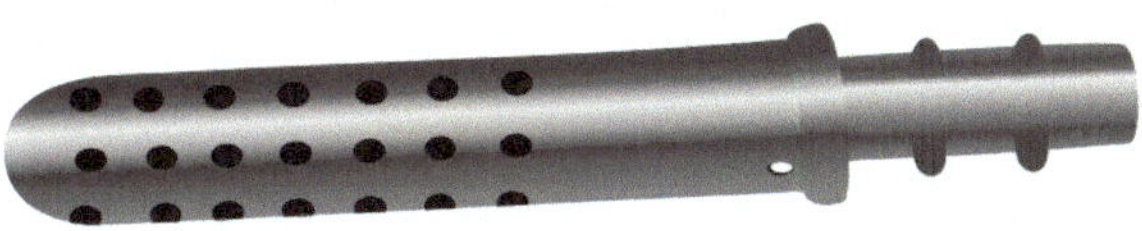

Adult
5 cm – 2"
Ped
3 cm – 1¼"
Bullet

Fig. 8.5: Young and pediatric bullet size

Uses

- It is connected to long catheter and used as a flexible vent
- To vent right and left atrium.

CHAPTER

9

Miscellaneous Instruments

MITRAL VALVE HOOK

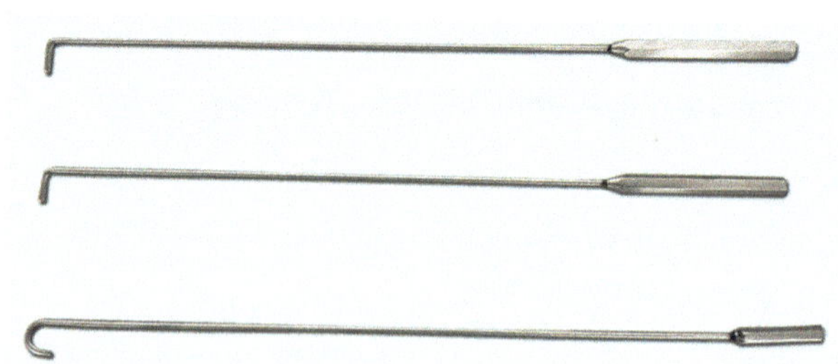

Fig. 9.1: Mitral valve hook

DeBakey Mitral Valve Hook

Special Feature

- Serration at hook for good grip (Fig. 9.1).

Uses

- Retraction of anterior and posterior mitral leaflets
- Check prolapse part of leaflet
- Check subvalvular structure

AORTIC PUNCH

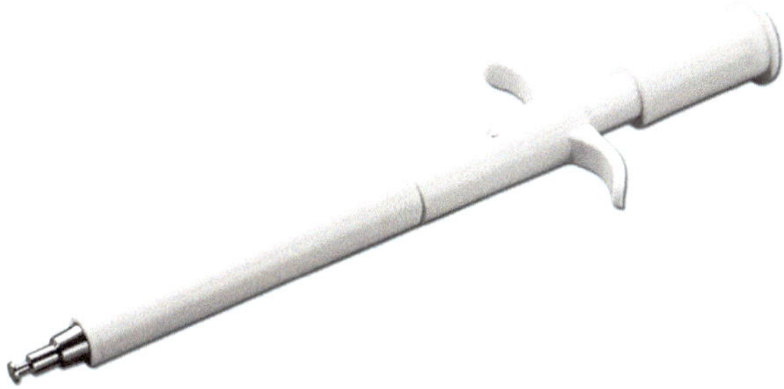

Fig. 9.2: Aortic punch

Specific Feature

- Disposable and reusable type available (Fig. 9.2)
- 3, 3.5, 4, 4.5 mm punch.

Uses

- Make hole in proximal ascending aorta for proximal anastomosis in CABG
- Make hole in aorta for central shunt proximal anastomosis
- Create a hole in neoaorta in arterial switch procedure to transfer coronary artery.

KARP AORTIC PUNCH OLD VERSION

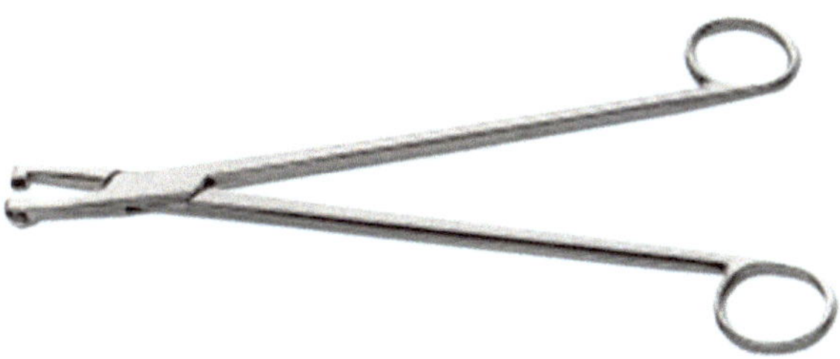

Fig. 9.3: Karp aortic punch

Advantage

This is a reusable instrument.

Disadvantage

Aortotomy requires to make hole.

SWEET STERNAL PUNCH

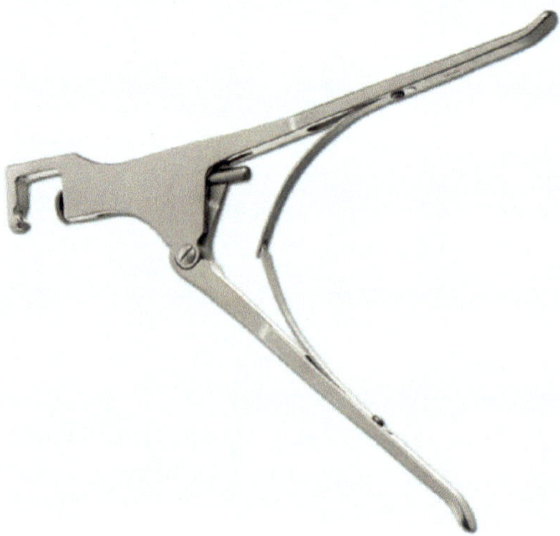

Fig. 9.4: Sweet sternal punch

Uses

Create hole in sternum so that sternal wires can be passed easily (Fig. 9.4).

STERNAL WIRE CUTTER

Uses

To cut twisted sternal wires (Fig. 9.5).

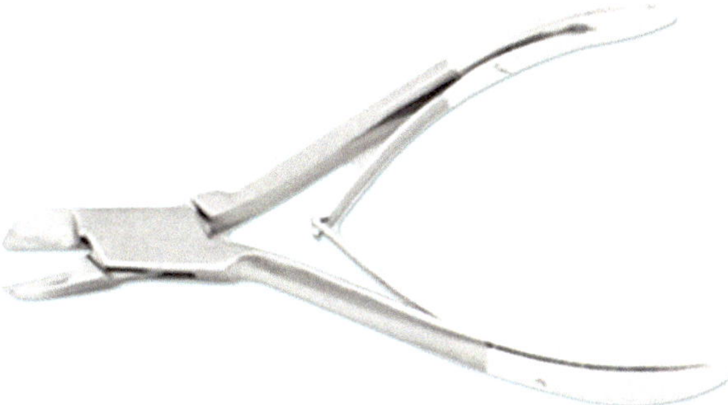

Fig. 9.5: Sternal wire cutter

RUMEL STYLET

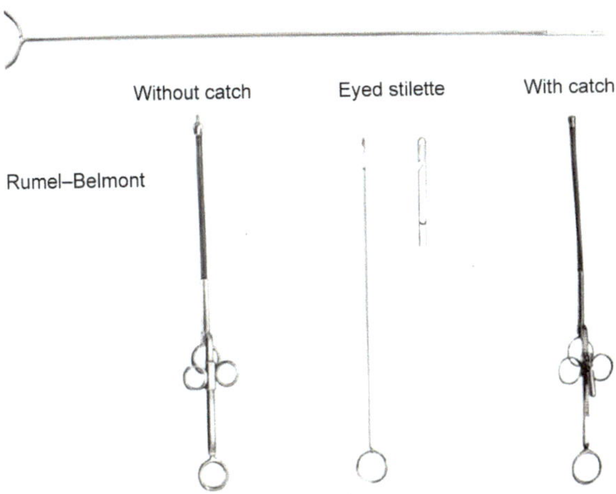

Fig. 9.6: Rumel stylet

Uses

To snare sutures or umbilical tape (Fig. 9.6).

CHAPTER

10

Instruments for off-pump CABG

TISSUE STABILIZERS

Octopus (Medtronic)

Uses

- Epicardial stabilizer for coronary artery anastomosis in off-pump and on-pump coronary artery bypass surgery (Fig. 10.1).

ACROBAT I STABILIZING SYSTEM (GUIDANT)

Figure 10.2 shows Acrobat I Stabilizing system.

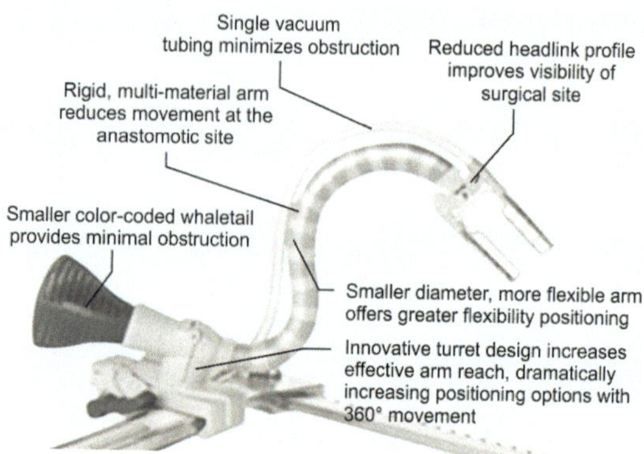

Fig. 10.1: Octopus tissue stabilizer

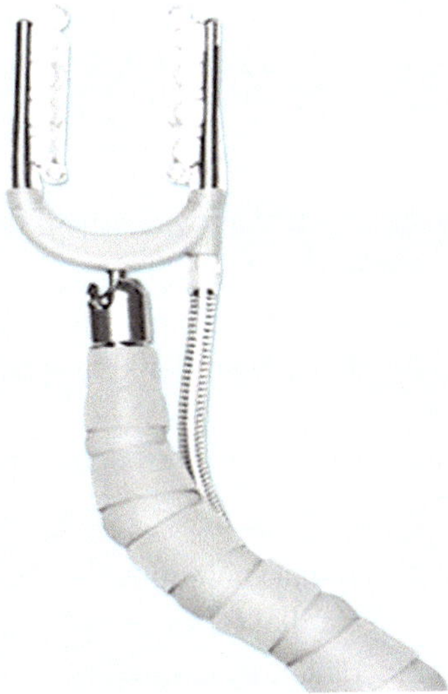

Fig. 10.2: Acrobat I Stabilizing system

STARFISH HEART POSITIONERS

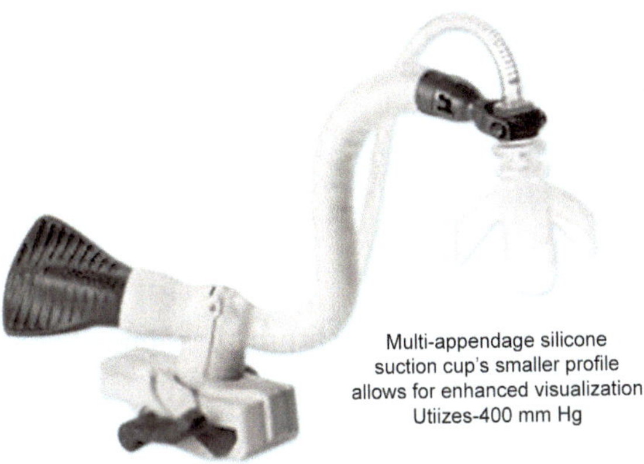

Fig. 10.3: Multi-appendage silicone suction cup-400 mm Hg

- Multiappendage silicon suction cup—400 mm Hg
- Flexible, low profile mounting with turret design.

Uses

- To lift heart apex, which provides good access to lateral wall for OM anastomosis
- Minimize hemodynamic deterioration with beating heart manipulation as it prevents kinking at RVOT site.

Q. Which are the other ways of Positioning Heart for Lateral Wall Anastomosis?

- Take deep pericardial stay suture at left side, pull it and fix it, and relax pericardial suture at right side
- Open right-sided pleura completely
- Head down and towards surgeon
- Place wet sponge below heart.

Q. Why Lateral Positioing can cause hemodynamic disturbance?

- Tilting heart on right side can obstruct main pulmonary artery flow which leads to low cardiac output
- Tilting can cause mitral regurgitation which lead to low cardiac output.

URCHIN HEART POSITIONER

- Silicon suction cup which provides immediate tissue capture, it utilizes—250 mm Hg suction pressure (Fig. 10.4).
- 360° movement
- Used for lateral wall anastomosis.

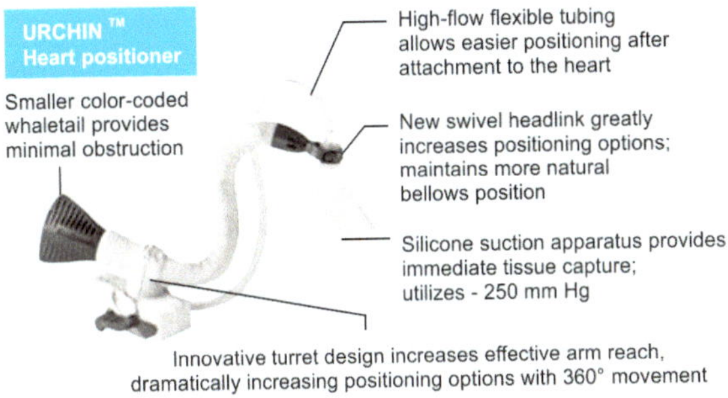

Fig. 10.4: Urchin heart positioner

SIMILAR PRODUCT

X-pose 4 from Maquet

X-pose 4 positioner can be placed on the heart apically or nonapically (Fig. 10.5).

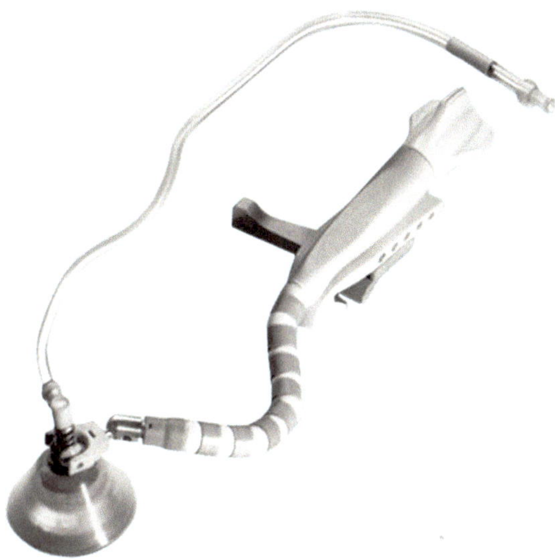

Fig. 10.5: X-pose 4 positioner

Starfish–NS Heart Positioner

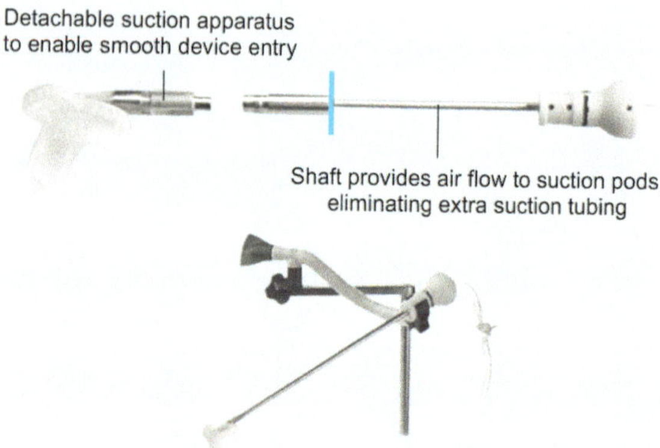

Fig. 10.6: Starfish—NS heart positioner

- It is a modification of original starfish positioner (Fig. 10.6)
- Detachable suction apparatus for smooth device entry from small incision
- Shaft provides air flow to pods eliminating extra suction tubing (Fig. 10.6).

Mist Blower

Method of Use

- Normal saline bottle should connect to saline port while gas port should be connected to CO_2 cylinder
- Regulate NS with regulator while CO_2 should be kept at 80–100
- Use of CO_2 is ideal to prevent air embolism.

Uses

- In beating heart CABG it provides bloodless field.

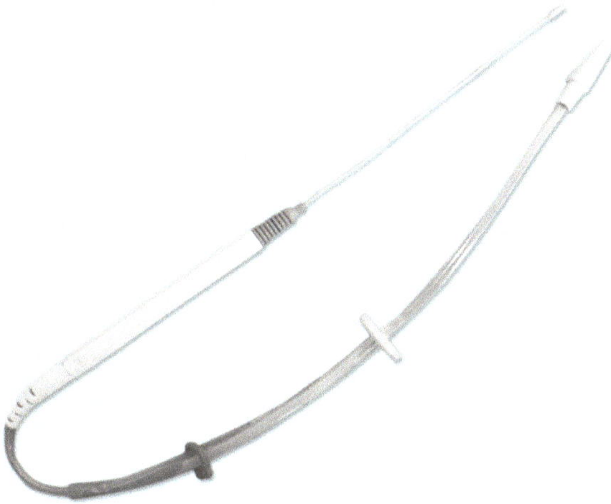

Fig. 10.7: Mist blower

ACROBAT-i Blower Mister Device

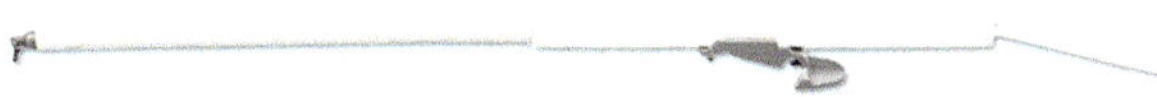

Fig. 10.8: Acrobat-I blower

- This is designed in such a way that shaft is malleable and handle is adjustable
- Its nozzle can be adjusted at proper point
- It is hands free, can be attached to retractor at proper position (Fig. 10.8).

INTRACORONARY SHUNTS

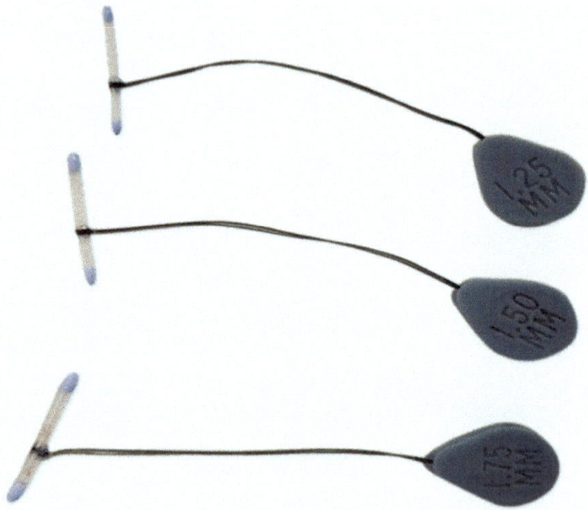

Fig. 10.9: Intracoronary shunts

Specification

- Soft with atraumatic tip, thread tied at center
- Different sizes available (Fig. 10.9).

Uses

- In beating heart CABG after arteriotomy, insertion of adequate size shunt maintain coronary flow distally and gives bloodless field
- Small size shunt comes out frequently and blood may leak sideways makes anastomosis difficult
- Larger size may not enter distally or snugly fit makes anastomosis difficult
- Sometimes, it can cause dissection of coronary artery also.

SPECIAL STERNAL RETRACTORS

Octobase (Metronic) Retractor

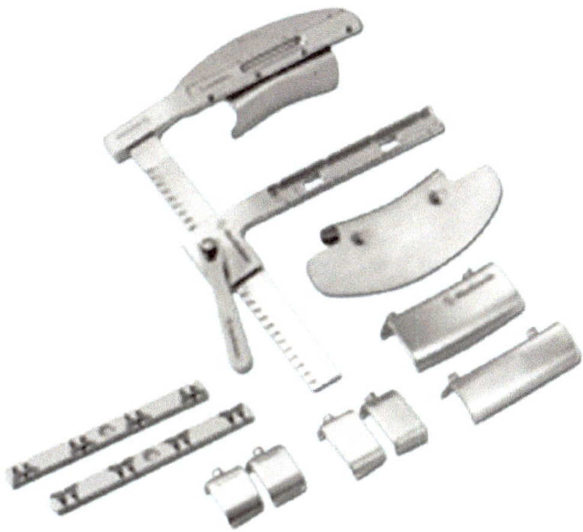

Fig. 10.10: Octobase sternal retractor

Acrobat (Guidant) Retractor

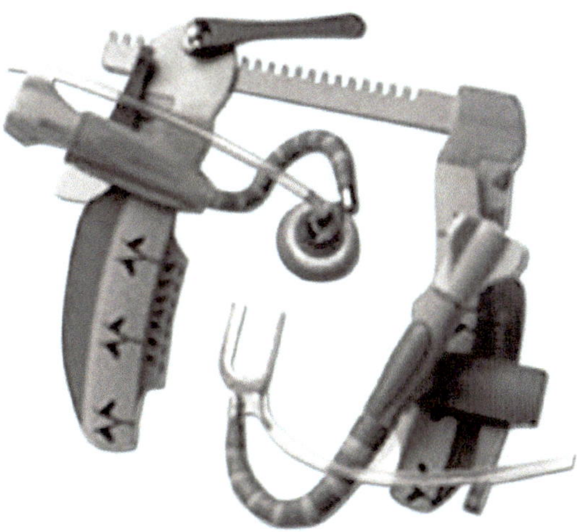

Fig. 10.11: Sternal retractor

This special retractor gives good attachment to the respective stabilizers and other accessories (Figs 10.10 and 10.11).

Epicardial Retractor (IMA)

Uses

- Retract extra epicardial fat for better distal anastomosis in CABG (Fig. 10.12)

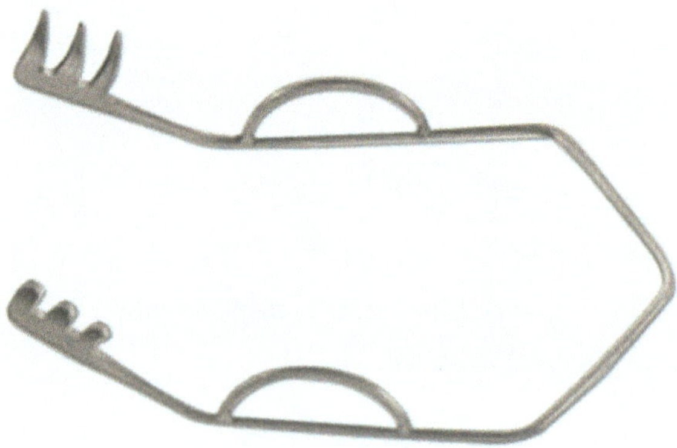

Fig. 10.12: Epicardial retractor

Other Methods of Retraction of Epicardial Fat

- Horizontal metress suture on either side helps to retract fat.

CHAPTER

11

Instrumentation for Minimally Invasive Cardiac Surgery

INTRODUCTION

Minimally invasive cardiac surgery (MICS) has been used since the early nineties; smaller incisions, robots and endoscopes were used by some pioneering surgeons to perform nearly every possible cardiac surgery; however, these techniques failed to achieve widespread popularity due to lack of training in this area, risk of fatal complication, excessive costs and prolonged procedure time. However, due to the greater effectiveness of interventional cardiology, surgeons have woken up to the fact that innovation is the need of the hour, and in collaboration with industry, several innovative devices and instruments have been designed to make MICS safer and cost effective.

MICS MITRAL VALVE SURGERY

Preoperative Set-up

The patient is positioned on a standard operating table with an inflatable cushion under the right scapula, an adequately sized sand bag under the scapula is another alternative, both groin and the sternum should be prepared and exposed for quick access in an emergency. External adhesive defibrillator paddles should be stuck in place, one on the right scapula and the other on the left lateral thoracic wall. Two arterial lines, one on the left radial and the other in the left femoral, should be placed. The central venous monitoring triple lumen catheter should be introduced via the left internal jugular vein, in cases where the right atrium is likely to be opened (ASD closure and tricuspid valve repairs). A double lumen endotracheal tube and transesophageal echocardiography with an experienced anesthetist are mandatory.

Operative Set-up

A high definition videomonitor and endoscopy system or Davinci Robotic system should be available in all cases. Most surgeons would use direct vision for most part of the surgical procedure; however, excellent illumination and visualization in critical steps, such as central aortic cannulation and cross clamping are done safely with video assistance (Fig. 11.1).

Incision for the procedures are primarily dictated by the patient's body habitus, but is commonly a 6–7 cm anterolateral incision running from the midclavicular line to the anterior axillary line (Fig. 11.2).

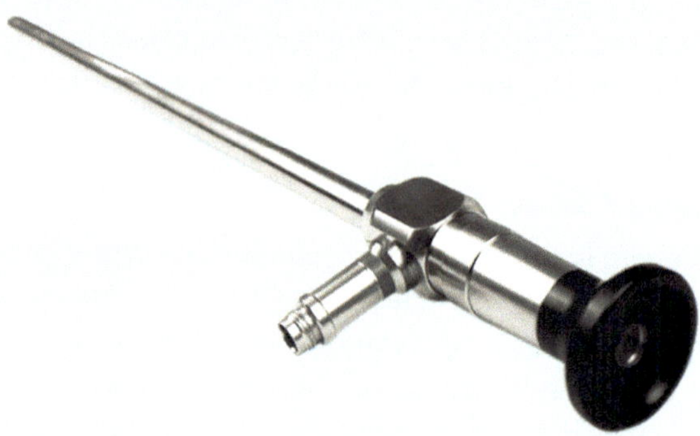

Fig. 11.1: Endoscope

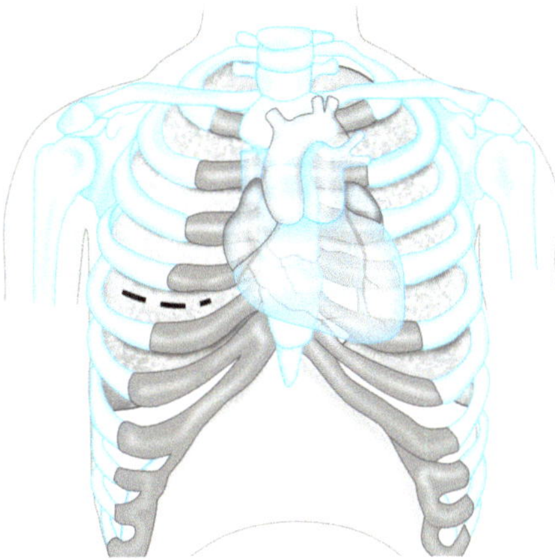

Fig. 11.2: Incision line

INSTRUMENTS

Soft Tissue Retractors

Soft tissue retractors are key to avoiding rib spreading, this will completely eliminate postoperative pain.

Alexis (Alexis O Wound Retractor, Applied Medical, Rancho Santa Margarita, CA, USA) soft tissue retractors are disposable soft tissue retractors. There are reusable soft tissue retractors from various companies that might reduce the cost of surgery.

Adhesive tapes around the incision will further reduce the soft tissue injury and improve exposure of the heart (Figs 11.3 and 11.4).

Tip: Partial resection of the fourth rib before application of the retractor will provide unparalleled exposure with minimal impact on postoperative pain, commonly the fourth or the fifth rib is partially resected.

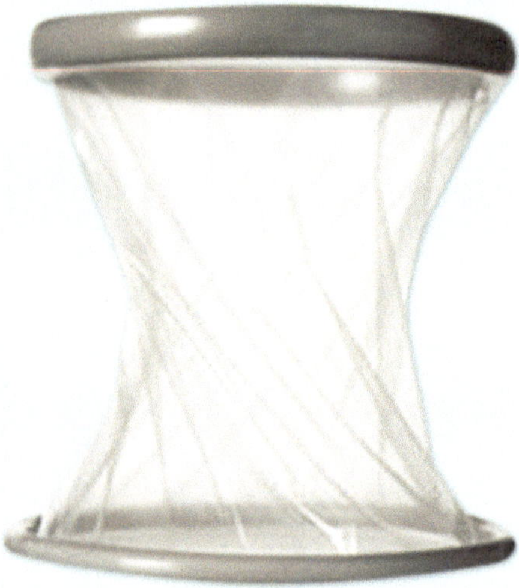

Fig. 11.3: Alexis wound retractor

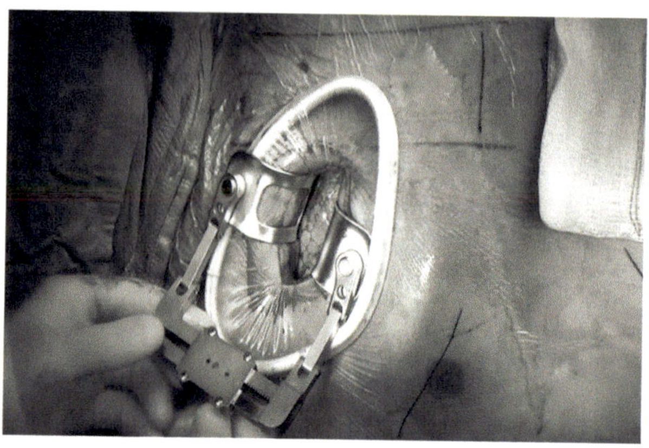

Fig. 11.4: Alexis wound retractor shown in use

Video Assistance

A 5 mm videothoracoscope, 30° angle is introduced through a 5 mm port in the 4th or 5th intercostal space in the space 2–3 cm posterior to the incision. A 10 mm port is introduced two space below in the posterior axillary line; stay sutures, CO_2 insufflation and graspers can be introduced through this port.

Cannulation

Arterial Cannulation

Both central and peripheral cannulation can be done according to surgeon preference and patients femoral artery status.

Many centers go in for percutaneous cannulation using the Seldinger technique; however, a 1–2 cm groin crease incision and a direct vision cannulation is preferable, as the femoral artery size, disease and cannula size can be accurately determined.

Several low resistance high flow cannulae are available for femoral arterial cannulation; however, innovative cannulas, such as the easy flow (estech, San Ramon, CA, USA), and the direct arterial cannula from Edwards could make central cannulation easier and safer for the patients. The direct arterial cannula comes with a pointed blade on the tip which makes central aortic cannulation bloodless and safe (Fig. 11.5).

Venous Cannula

Peripheral femoral venous cannulation avoids extra cannula in the incision and allows for better access to perform surgery; however, some centers routinely cannulate the right internal

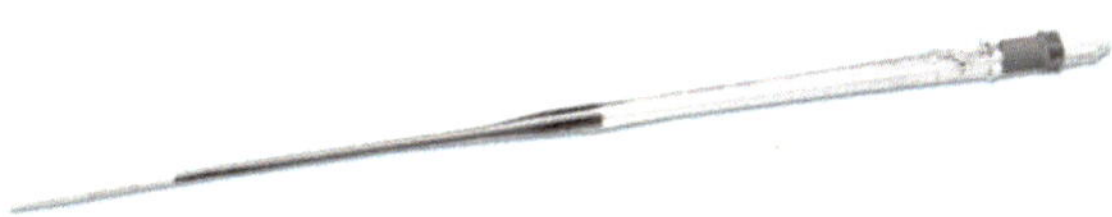

Fig. 11.5: Arterial cannula

jugular vein. The Edwards quick draw venous cannulas and the multistage biomedicus cannulas from Medtronic (Minneapolis, MN, USA) have obviated the need for separate superior caval cannulae,when working through the left atrium. These cannulae can be used in right atrial operations when positioned correctly with TOE guidance (Fig. 11.6). Using suction device to improve venous drainage can be useful in some patients.

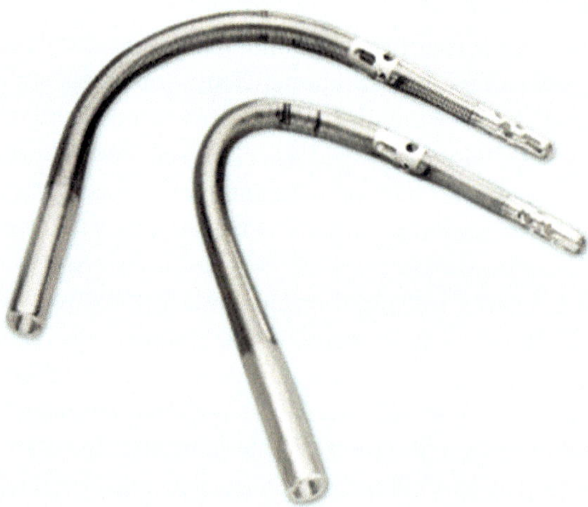

Fig. 11.6: Venous cannula

MYOCARDIAL PROTECTION

Most centers prefer to use retrograde coronary perfusion as the only means of protection or in conjunction with antegrade cardioplegia delivered through the root.

Retrograde cannulation can be done through a purse- string suture parallel to and 2 cm below the atrioventricular groove. TOE guidance is mandatory as coronary sinus injury can be devastating.

Aortic Crossclamp

Aortic crossclamping is one of the most critical steps of the operation. Some centers prefer an endoclamp, that is passed through the femoral artery and positioned in the ascending aorta, this is inflatable balloon and can occlude aortas with diameters up to 35 mm. Cardioplegia can be administered through the central lumen (Figs 11.7).

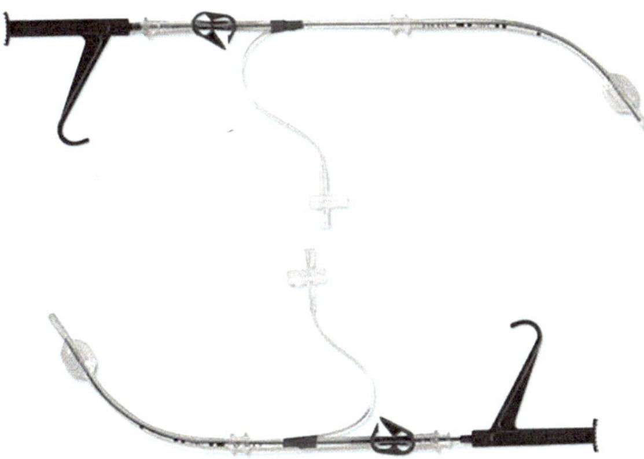

Fig. 11.7: Retrograde cardioplegia cannula

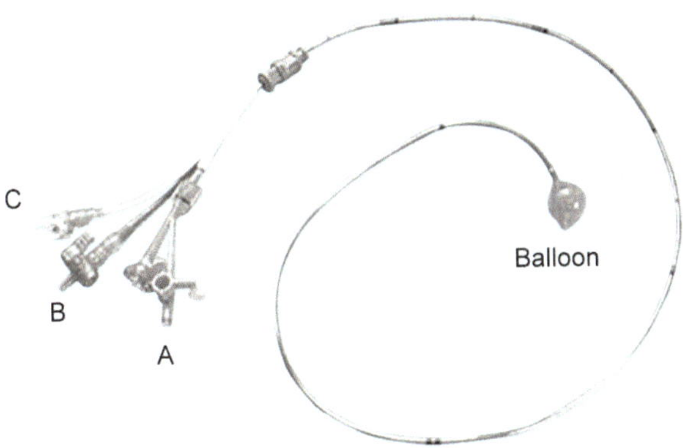

Fig. 11.8: Balloon inflatable endoclamp

However, most centers would prefer a transthoracic Chitwood DeBakey that can be passed through a stab incision in the midclavicular line or through the second space anteriorly (Fig. 11.9).

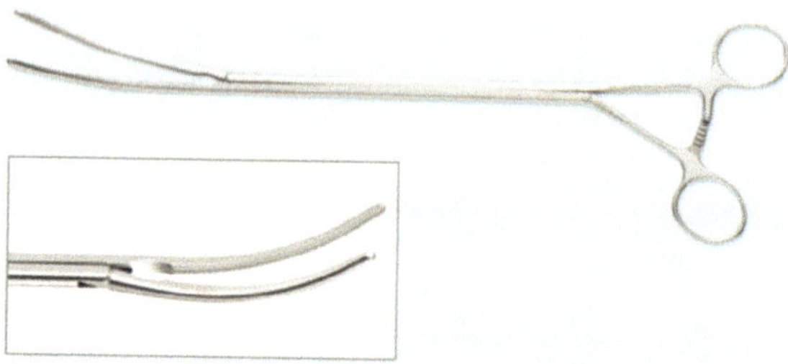

Fig. 11.9: Chitwood DeBakey clamp

However, recently, there are several new clamps that are flexible and can be safely applied through the incision and avoid cutting in the operating field (Fig. 11.10).

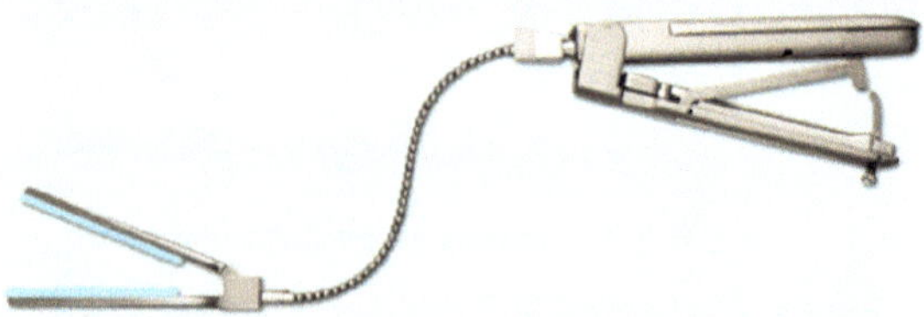

Fig. 11.10: Aortic crossclamp shown with ultra-insert

SPECIAL INSTRUMENTS

Atrial Retractors

A variety of retractors have been developed by various companies to give excellent exposure of the mitral valve.

Intercostal retractor with blades of various sizes are available that can be interchanged according to the patients body habitus.

A selection of left atrial retractors that are specifically designed to retract the atrial roof, can be either malleable or rigid. They also come in various sizes and shapes (Figs 11.11A to C).

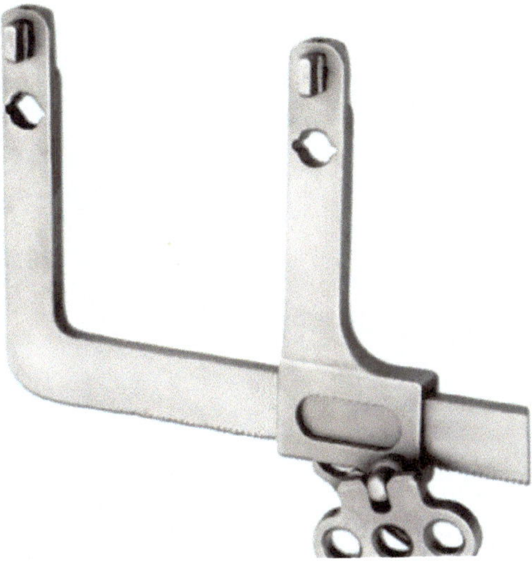

A

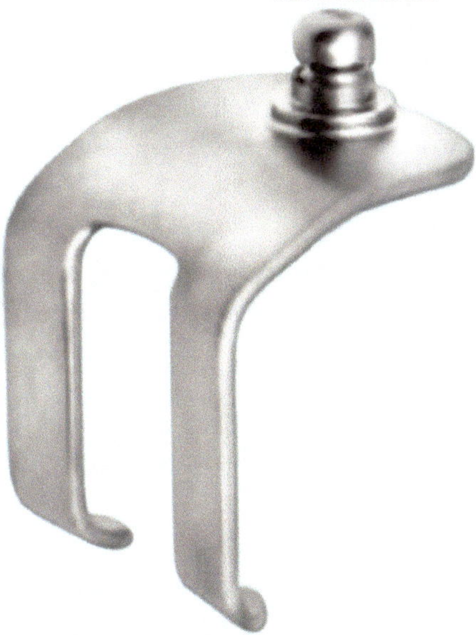

B

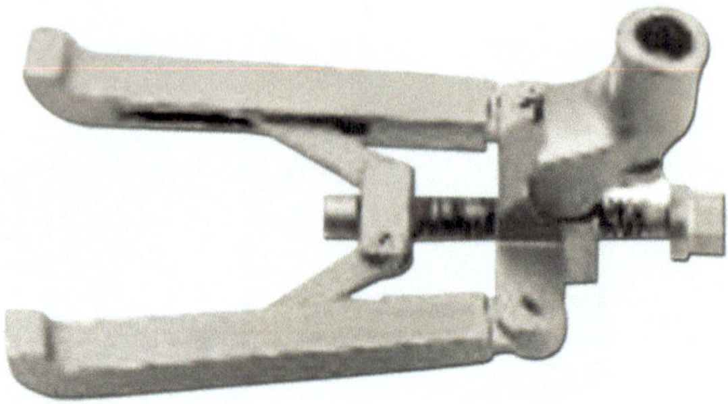

C

Figs 11.11A to C: Left atrial retractor

These retractors provide a clutter free operating field, where minor adjustments to the type of blades and their angle provides excellent exposure. It may take up a few minutes to set up the retractor and obtain the perfect exposure, this is time consuming.

The assistants hands are freed, and operating field must not be obstructed.

TIP

It is important to have retrograde cardioplegia as it would be difficult to take down the system to give repeated antegrade CP.

MICS MITRAL INSTRUMENTS

Minimally invasive rib spreader with attachments are available.

MICS Needle Holder

Needle holders, typically, are made of stainless steel (light-weight ones made up of other material are also available). They come with a straight or curved tip in various jaw sizes. The shaft is usually 30–35 cm long, and can be chosen according to chest cavity depth and surgeon preference. The action is

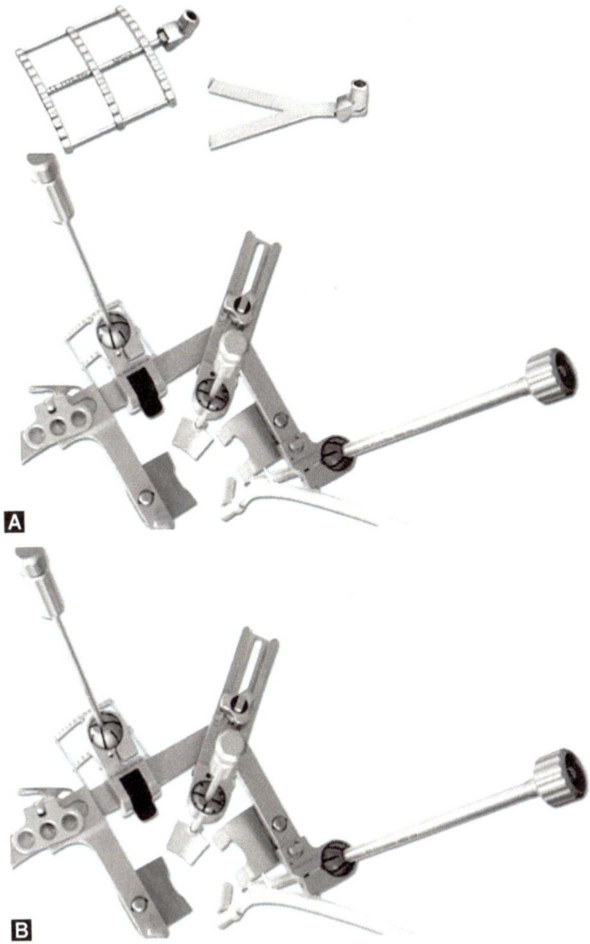

Figs 11.12A and B: Rib retractors provide excellent exposure

usually a round squeeze handle, with textured grips. Ratcheted and non-ratcheted needle holders are available according to surgeon preference.

MICS Scissors

MICS scissors are available at different lengths ranging from 30 to 35 cm, they also come with a straight, curved and strongly curved working ends, like the needle drivers they also have a squeeze angle.

MICS Forceps

MICS forceps with DeBakey serration are standard and are invaluable.

Atraumatic jaws that are invaluable in manipulating the atria and pacing purse-strings in the aorta, superior vena cava and making incisions on the heart and also grasping fine needles 30–35 cm, allowing adequate reach.

- Curved and straight jaws (Figs 11.13A and B)
- Convenient squeeze action
- With or without ratchets.

MICS Resano Forceps and Serrated Edges

These forceps are used to grasp valve tissue, aiding in mitral repairs and replacements, the curved scissors are useful in resecting the anterior leaflet in replacements and the serrated ones are useful in holding leaflet tissue.

- 30–35 cm in length
- Convenient and easy-to-use squeeze handles.

MICS Russian Forceps and Biopsy Forceps

As in the normal forceps, these forceps are used in clearing left atrial clot, decalcifying the annulus and leaflet.

- 35 cm in length
- Rounded squeeze handles
- Invaluable in tying knots when working at depth.

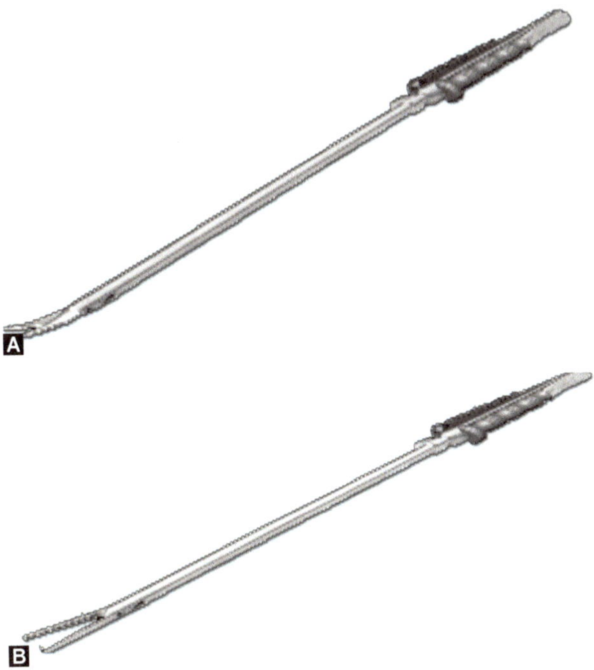

Figs 11.13A and B: MICS forceps. (A) Curved jaw; (B) Straight jaw

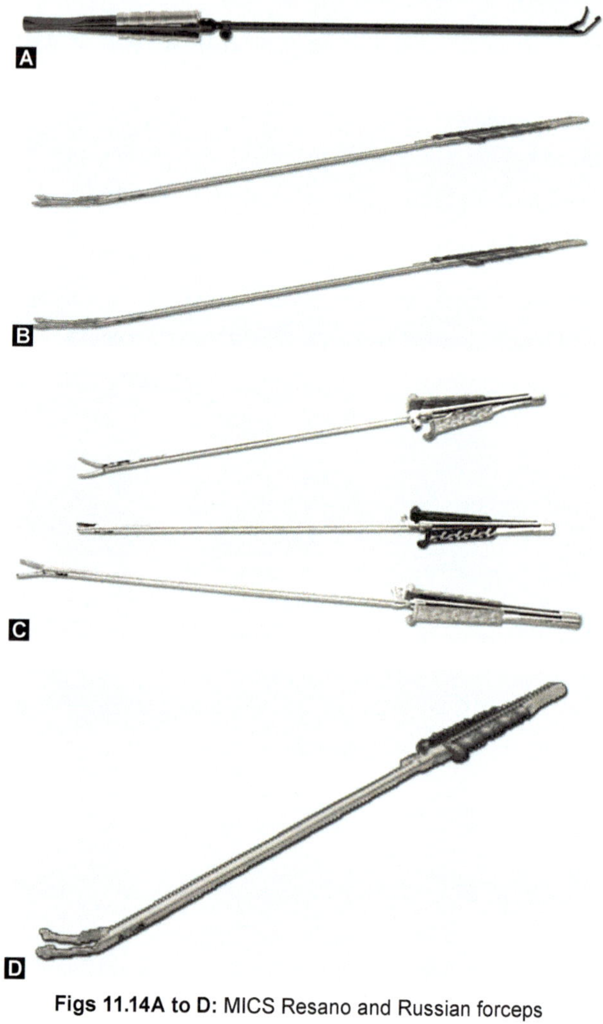

Figs 11.14A to D: MICS Resano and Russian forceps

MICS Knot Pusher

There are two commonly used types from Edwards Inc and Fehling Instruments. This instrument is essential to tie down knots at depth during mitral valve surgery. Adequate training in the use of this instrument is required before use to avoid loose sutures.

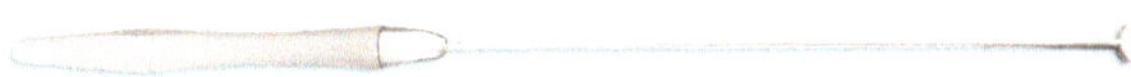

Fig. 11.15: MICS knot pusher

OTHER USEFUL INSTRUMENTS

Minimally invasive clip applicator, hooks, suture pullers, scalpel blade holders and suction tips.

Mitral surgery when done through a lower mid sternotomy can be done with standard instruments.

Instruments Required to do a MMICS Mitral Surgery through a Minithoracotomy

- Minimally invasive rib retractor system
- Flexible aortic cross clamp or a Chitwood type transthoracic aortic clamp
- Minimal invasive suture puller
- Left atrial retractor
- Minimally invasive scissors, curved
- Minimally invasive scissors, 30°
- Minimally invasive knot pusher
- Minimally invasive needle drivers

- Minimally invasive forceps straight
- Forceps Resano type
- Minimally invasive hook.

MINIMALLY INVASIVE CORONARY ARTERY BYPASS SURGERY

MICS Retractor System

- Octopus® Nuvo Stabilizer
- Starfish® NS Positioner
- U-CLIP® Anastomotic Device
- Mounting System for Octopus® Nuvo and Starfish® NS
- R ultract® with Skyhook Retractor
- Small and Medium Endoscopic Clip Appliers
- Knot Pusher
- Minimally Invasive (MI) Needle Holder
- Minimally Invasive Curved Scissors
- Minimally Invasive Debakey Forceps
- Tangential Occlusion Clamp
- DeBakey Aorta Clamp—Full Curved DeBakey
- Soft Tissue Retractor
- Extended Bovie Blade

The Octopus® Nuvo Tissue Stabilizer Features

- Low profile Octopus tissue stabilizer
- Smaller, 3-pod head
- Malleable pods for flexibility
- Detachable head with quick-connect for remote shaft insertion and attachment
- Increased flexibility to aid positioning
- Usually inserted though the sixth space access incision and can be held in place by a specially designed crossbar that fits onto the operating table (Fig. 11.16).

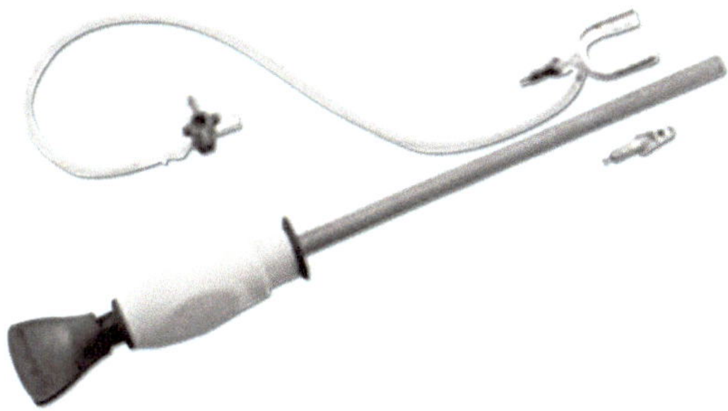

Fig. 11.16: Tissue stabilizer

THE STARFISH POSITIONER

The features are as follows (Fig. 11.17).

- Detachable suction head
- Presents coronary arteries for direct vision anastomosis
- Does not clutter the surgical field and is inserted through a small stab incision at the level of the xiphoid bone

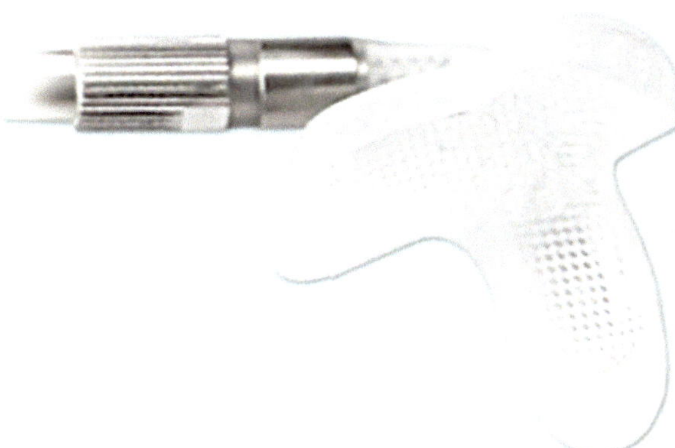

Fig. 11.17: The starfish positioner

- Using the starfish positioner all the coronary arteries can be accessed by small manipulation without hemodynamic compromise (Fig. 11.18)
- MICS retractor system with lift blades, these blades are fixed to a crossbar attachment (skyhook) that goes onto the operating table and the chest wall is 'lifted' to aid in harvest of the internal thoracic artery
- Good access can be gained to safely harvest from the fifth to the first intercostal space.

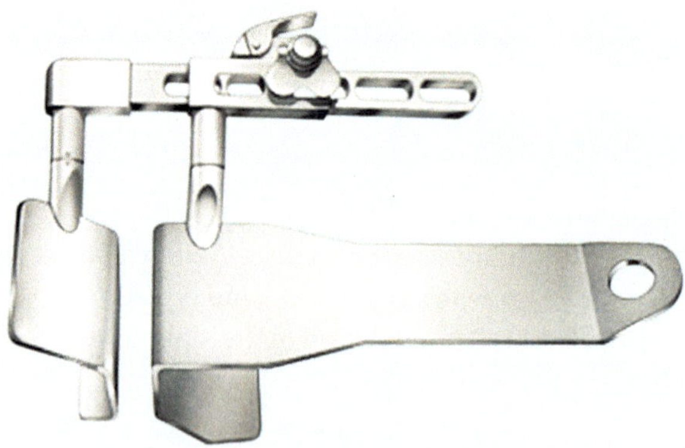

Fig. 11.18: All the coronary arteries can be accessed using the starfish positioner

MINIMALLY INVASIVE AORTIC VALVE SURGERY

This procedure is performed through a right mini thoracotomy incising the pleura along the 2nd or 3rd right intercostal space or through a upper ministernotomy.

Minimally Invasive AVR through upper hemisternotomy can be performed in most patients with standard instruments and a soft tissue MICS retractor.

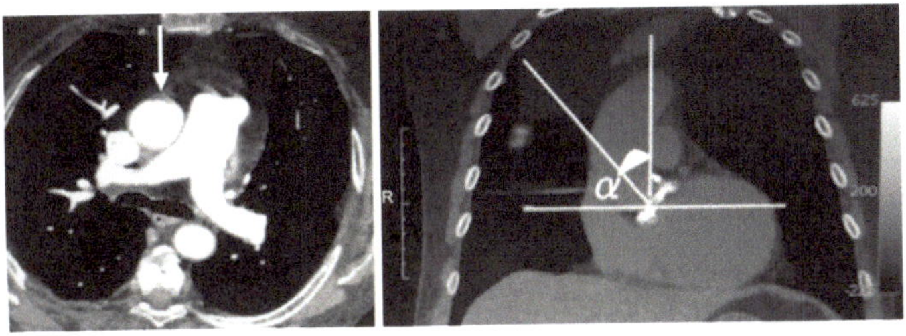

Fig. 11.19: CT evaluation

Minimally Invasive AVR through right mini thoracotomy can be offered to selected group of patients after performing a Noncontrast Chest CT scan to assess the lie of the aorta and angle of the aortic root. The aorta should be rightward with 50% lateral to the right sternal border, ascending aorta should be less than 10 cm from the sternum and the angle of the alpha angle of the aortic root should be greater than 45 Degrees (Fig. 11.19).

CHAPTER

12

Sutures and Needle

The word suture describes any strands of materials used to ligate blood vessels or approximate tissue to close the wound.

IDEAL SUTURES

- Minimal tissue reaction
- Easy to handle
- Easy to knot
- High tensile strength
- Smooth passage through the tissue
- Consistent performance.

CLASSIFICATION OF SUTURES

- Sutures are classified depending upon its different properties:
    - Absorbable Or Nonabsorbable
    - Monofilament Or Braided
    - Synthetic Or Natural

Absorbable Sutures

- Absorbable sutures are made of material which are broken down in tissues after a given period of time
- Depending on the material it can be absorbed in tissues from 10 days to 8 weeks.

- As the suture is absorbed by the body tissues within three week's time, therefore, no need for the patient to have the suture removal
- Absorbable sutures are made from gut mucosa or synthetic polymer fibers which may be braided or monofilament
- Synthetic absorbable offers numerous advantages over gut sutures, notably ease of handling, low cost, low tissue reaction, etc.

Natural Absorbable Suture

These are originally made up of intestines of sheep, the so called catgut.

- Treated with formaldehyde
- Chromic catgut: treated with chromic salt
- Increases strength
- Slow loss of tensile strength
- Decreases tissue reaction
- Absorbed by phagocytosis
- Rapidly absorbable
- Loses tensile strength (33% in 7 days, 67% in 28 days)
- Broken down within a week.

Advantages

- Relatively good handling characteristics
- Stiff in larger sizes
- Good knot security
- Chromic acid delays hydrolysis
- Catgut has been replaced by synthetic absorbable polymers.

Characters

- Natural
- Rapidly absorbable
- Multifilament

Disadvantages

- Tend to induce more tissue reaction than synthetic material.

Types of Absorbable and Nonabsorbable Sutures

Absorbable sutures include the following:
- *Polyglycolic acid sutures*
- *Polyglactin 910*
- *Catgut*
- *Polyglecaprone 25*
- *Polydioxanone sutures.*

Nonabsorbable sutures include the following:
- *Polypropylene sutures*
- *Nylon (polyamide)*
- *Polyester*
- *Silk*
- *Stainless steel sutures.*

Synthetic Absorbable Sutures

Synthetic absorbable sutures offer the strength needed for a wide range of applications, from abdominal and chest wound closure to ophthalmic and plastic surgery.

Nowadays, synthetic suture material is the type most widely used.

Synthetic sutures have replaced natural sutures because they offer improved tolerance and a more predictable resorption profile in case of absorbable sutures.

Advantages

- Minimal tissue reaction
- Absorption by hydrolysis

- Tensile strength retention 28–35 days
- Tend to lose tensile strength and are absorbed at more predictable rate
- Common examples include polydioxanone (PDS).

NONABSORBABLE SUTURE

Those sutures which are not digested by body enzymes or hydrolyzed in body tissues are called nonabsorbable sutures.

They are made from a variety of non biodegradable materials and are ultimately encapsulated or walled off by the body's fibroblasts. Nonabsorbable sutures ordinarily remain where they are burried within the tissues.

1. Silk sutures—black braided suture
2. Polypropylene sutures (Prolene)—monofilament suture
3. Nylon suture or polyamide sutures—monofilament suture
4. Polyester sutures—coated and braided suture.

Natural Nonabsorbable Sutures

- Silk sutures
- Cotton sutures
- Linen sutures.

Surgical Silk Black Braided

- Most widely used nonabsorbable suture
- Very pliable and easy to knot
- Braided high knot security
- Suture: silk
- Color: black
- Construction: braided
- Absorption: nonabsorbable.

Commonly used to tie in surgical drains, repair small holes in the bowel or tie off large blood vessels.

Synthetic Nonabsorbable

- Polypropylene sutures
- Polyamide monofilament sutures
- Coated braided polyester suture
- Stainless steel suture.

Advantages of Synthetic Nonabsorbable Sutures

- Very high tensile strength
- Consistent performance
- Virtually non-biodegradable
- Extremely nonreactive.

Monofilament-Nonabsorbable Sutures

Monofilament surgical sutures are made of a single strand. This structure is relatively more resistant to harboring micro-organisms. The monofilament sutures exhibit less resistance to passage through tissue than multifilament suture. Great care must be taken in handling and tying monofilament suture because crushing or crimping of this suture can nick or weaken the suture and lead to undesirable and premature suture failure.

Suture Name—Prolene

- Construction—Monofilament
- Absorption—Nonabsorbable
- Color—Clear or blue

Prolene sutures often come double armed. This allows a surgeon to create an anastomosis with vascular grafts.

Ethilon is a synthetic nonabsorbable nylon suture manufactured by Ethicon. Black in color, it is a monofilament suture that is used frequently for soft-tissue approximation and ligation.

Even though it is nonabsorbable, the knot security decreases over time *(in vivo)* and should not be used where permanent retention is required.

PTFE Sutures

Strands of expanded PTFE.

Uses in Cardiac Surgery

- Vascular graft anastomosis mainly PTFE graft as it prevents needle hole bleeding
- Neochordal formation in case of mitral valve repair surgery
- Suspension suture for aortic valve repair in cusp prolapse.

Suture Materials Vary in their Physical Characteristics

- Monofilament sutures (e.g. polypropylene) are smooth
- They slide well in tissues but if handled inappropriately they can fracture.

Advantages

- Have less drag than multifilament suture
- Smooth surface, allows easy passage through tissue and noncapillary action
- Has no interstices to support bacterial growth.

Disadvantages

- With thicker threads renders knot-tying becomes more difficult

- Care should be taken in handling because any nick or damage with forceps or needle holder weakens them and predispose them to breakage.

MULTIFILAMENT NONABSORBABLE SUTURES

- *Polyester, silk*
- ***Polyester sutures used in cardiac surgery***
- *Aortic pursestring*
- *Atrial and caval pursestring*
- *Valve replacement*
- ***Use of silk in cardiac surgery***
- *Stay suture*
- *Ligation of vessels*
- *Drain fixation*
- *Pericardial stay.*

Multifilament Absorbable Sutures

Multifilament consist of several filaments or strands, twisted or braided together. This affords greater tensile strength, pliability, and flexibility. This type of suture handles and ties well. Because multifilament materials have increased capillarity, the increased absorption of fluid may act as a tract for the introduction of pathogens.

Multifilament Sutures (e.g. Polyglactin) are Braided

- They have a greater surface area
- They are easier to handle and knot well.

Advantages

- Consists of several fibers twisted or braided into a single strand
- Generally stronger
- Usually better knot security

- More tissue drag
- Many available with coatings applied by manufacturer to minimize tissue drag but also decreases knot security
- Should not be placed in infected or contaminated areas
- Multifilament sutures are more pliable and flexible than monofilament sutures
- Results in considerably better knot holding security
- Better handling
- Tight weaving of multifilament sutures provide minimum friction.

Disadvantages

- Longitudinal orientation of the individual filaments within the thread results in relatively high capillarity, but the capillarity of braided threads is less than that of twisted threads.
- Multifilament sutures have a rough surface that impairs passage through tissue during surgical procedure
- Bacteria can reside between individual fibers of the strand
- Isolated from immune system and antibiotics
- Results in persistence of infection as long as suture present.

NEEDLES

The ideal surgical needle is made of high quality stainless steel as slim as possible without compromising strength, stable in the grasp of a needle holder, able to carry suture material through tissue with minimal trauma. Sharp enough to penetrate tissue with minimal resistance, rigid enough to resist bending but not break, steril and corrosion resistant.

Shapes

Shapes vary from straight to curved (Fig. 12.1).

- **Straight needles**

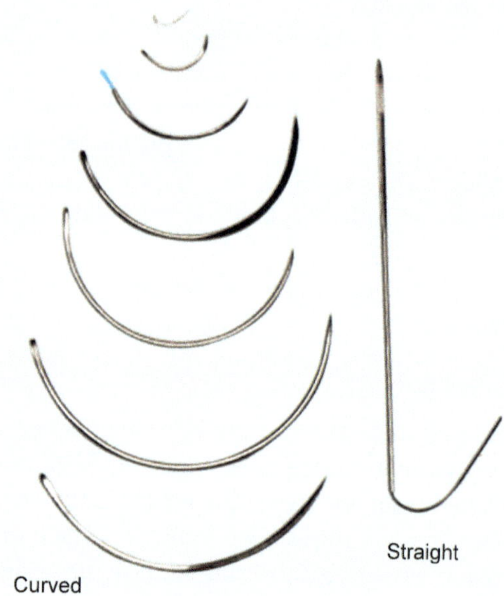

Fig. 12.1: Curved and straight needles

- Used near surface (primarily skin)
- Inserted through tissues with fingers not needle holders
- Usually combined with hand ties.

❑ **Curved needles**

- Manipulated with needle holders
- Rotating wrist in arc similar to that of needle is easiest and most efficient
- Curvature is described by amount of the circumference of a circle (e.g. 1/4, 3/8, 1/2, 5/8, etc.)
- Most common curves are 3/8 and 1/2
- Wider curves useful when suturing thick tissues or in deep or poorly accessible locations (easier to retrieve tip)
- Most commonly used.

NEEDLE TYPES

- Eyed
- Eyeless or swaged

Eyed Needle

- Suture threaded through eye during surgery from inside curve toward outside (Fig. 12.2)
- Reusable
- Economical
- Mainly used for suturing skin.

Disadvantages

- Less sharp if reused
- Less efficient (time spent threading needle)
- More traumatic (bigger hole because double strand of suture pulled through tissue)
- Avoid threading eye twice to prevent suture pulling out as it creates more tissue trauma.

Uses of Eyed Needle in Cardiac Surgery

- Used for pericardial stay
- Fixing of intercostal drainage.

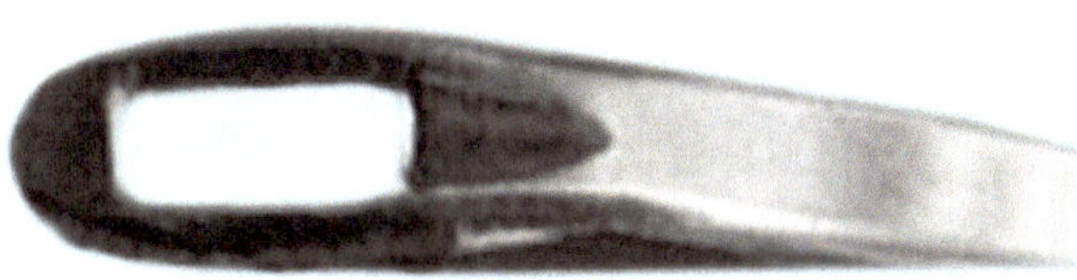

Fig. 12.2: Eyed needle

Eyeless Needle

- Suture permanently attached to the needle
- Consistently sharp with known shape and durability (not damaged by previous use)
- Convenient as threading not required (Fig. 12.3)
- More efficient as suture does not pull out while suturing
- Generally preferred.

Advantages

- Eyeless needle is composed of a single use needle and suture. This avoids the loss of sharpness that occurs with reusable needles
- There is only a single strand of suture that is pulled through the tissues, and the gap that is created by the needle is fully plugged by the suture. This reduces potential leakage through the suture line
- There is no rethreading of an eyeless needle
- Its use is more time efficient.

SIZE OF THE NEEDLE

- Needles come in various lengths and diameter
- Tissue to be sutured (larger for thick dense tissue, smaller for delicate tissue)

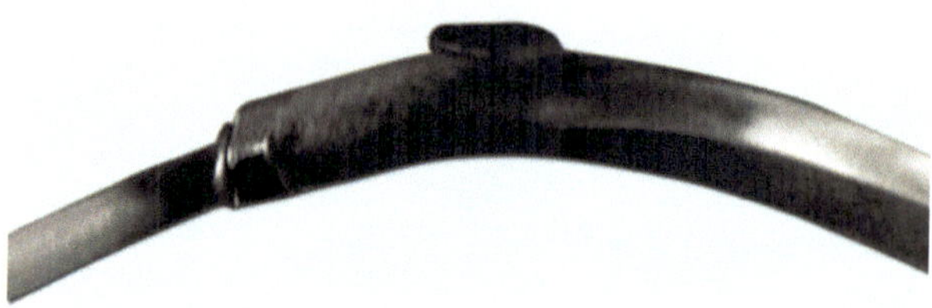

Fig. 12.3: Eyeless needle

- Size and location of wound
- Size of suture material needed to support incision during healing (bigger needle for larger suture

Selected needle should be (Fig. 12.4):

- Smallest that will do the job (minimize tissue trauma)
- Large enough not to bend during insertion or extraction
- Long enough to reach both sides of incision in a single pass

NEEDLE TYPES

Needles can be arranged into groups according to the design of the point.

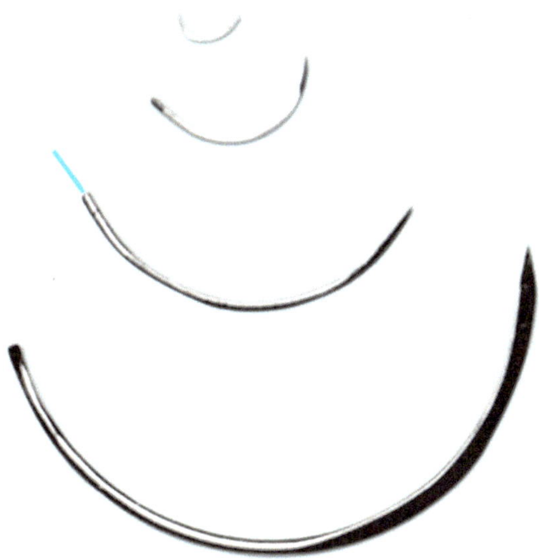

Fig. 12.4: Size of the needles

- The first group is round-bodied needles—a group with many modified variants
- The second group is cutting needles which are used in areas of tough or dense tissue and for suturing skin
- The third group is used mainly in ophthalmology and is of side cutting or spatulated point design.

I. Round bodied needle

- Blunt point needle
- Taper point
- Taper point plus
- CC needle
- Taper cut.

II. Cutting needle

- Reverse cutting
- Conventional cutting
- Trocar point.

Round-bodied Needle

- Round-bodied needles are designed to separate tissue fibers rather than cut them
- They are used either for soft tissue or in situations where easy splitting of tissue fibers is possible. After the passage of the needle, the tissue closes tightly round the suture material, thereby forming a leak-proof suture line which is particularly vital in intestinal and cardiovascular surgery
- Round-bodied needles are manufactured with different wire diameters according to the tissue to be sutured
- For softer tissue, such as bowel, finer wire diameters can be used
- Whereas for muscle or fascia heavier wire diameters are required.

Taper Point or Noncutting Needle

- Have a round body with a sharp pointed tip
- Generally used for viscera, muscle and light fascia
- Penetrates tissue, without cutting, creating a round holle.

Disadvantage

Should **NOT** be used for dense tissue like skin because the extraforce needed to penetrate the tissue causes extratrauma or bends the needle.

- **Taper cut tip** a newer design that combines the round body with a cutting tip so can be used for both delicate and dense tissue (Fig. 12.5)

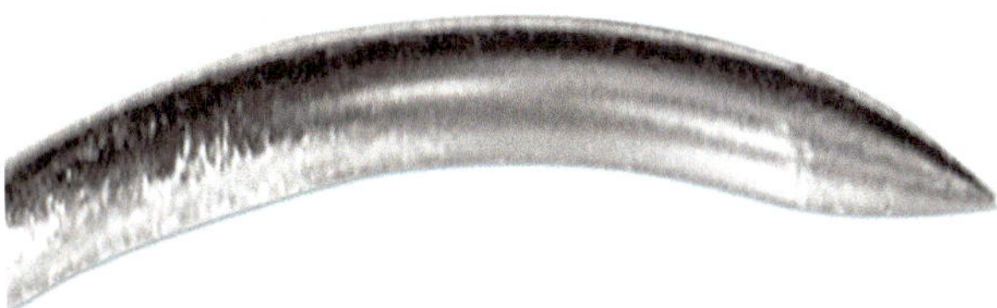

Fig. 12.5: Taper point

Visi-Black Needle

- These black needles have been designed to give outstanding visibility against tissue and where blood is present in the operating field
- The slim taper point design of the Visi-black needle brings improved penetration properties and minimizes tissue trauma.

Blunt Point Needle (Fig. 12.6)

- The needles has been designed to minimize the risk of needle stick injury
- The needle point is sharp enough to penetrate fascia and muscle but not skin
- Virtually eliminating accidental glove puncture; the needle can also be used for suturing friable tissue such as the liver
- This needle has been designed for suturing extremely friable tissue, such as the liver.

Advantages

Blunt nosed to dissect fragile tissue.

CC Needle

- The unique point design of the CC needle provides significantly improved penetration properties for the cardiac/vascular surgeon when suturing tough, calcified vessels
- This is achieved with no increase in tissue trauma compared to the conventional round bodied needle. Squared body

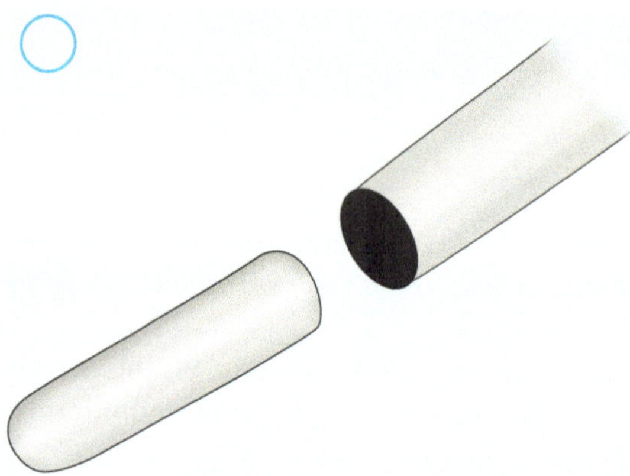

Fig. 12.6: Blunt point

geometry, in addition to providing a stronger fine vascular needle, also means this needle is particularly secure in the needle holder.

Tapercut Needle

- Easy penetration with minimized trauma.

Advantages

- Sharp gradually tapered needles guarantees easy penetration in every bite.

Cutting Needle for Fibrous Tissues

- Triangular shaped point with 2–3 cutting edges to facilitate penetration of dense tissue
- Cutting edge is on the inside of the curve (concave surface)
- **Cut edge is where the tension is on the tied suture so this type of needle predisposes the suture to cutting through the tissue (Fig. 12.7)**

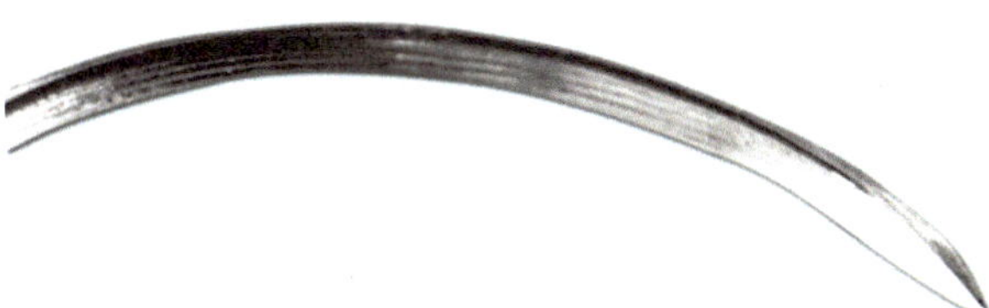

Fig. 12.7: Cutting needle for fibrous tissue

- Use has generally been replaced by the reverse cutting needle
- Cutting needles are required wherever fibrous or dense tissue needs to be sutured.

Reverse Cutting Needle

The body of this needle is triangular in cross section, having the apex cutting edge on the outside of the needle curvature. This improves the strength of the needle and particularly increases its resistance to bending. This is preferred by most surgeons (Fig. 12.8).

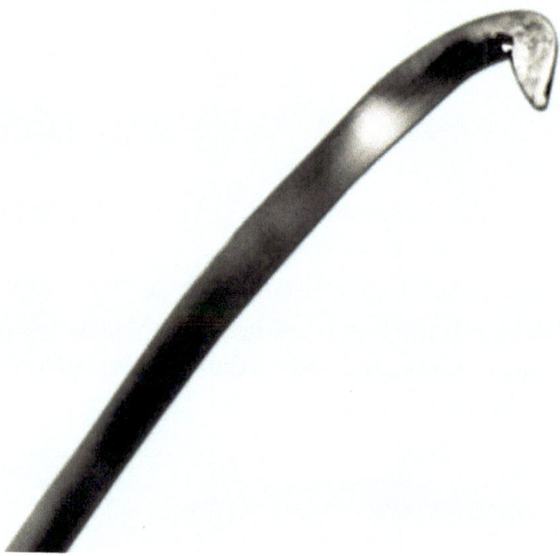

Fig. 12.8: Reverse cutting needle

Advantages

Accurately sharped 3 sides, easily cuts through dense, thick and difficult to penetrate tissue.

Trocar Point Needle

This trocar point cutting needles ensures powerful penetration, even when deep and dense tissue.

Cutting Needle for Skin Closure

Prime Needle

- The cross sectional geometry of the needle tip reduces the angles of the cutting edges which gives improved penetration and control
- A square body on the needle greatly increases needle strength and offers improved stability in the needle holder
- Prime needles are available with either a reverse cutting or a conventional cutting profile.

Conventional Cutting Needle

This needle has a triangular cross section with the apex of the triangle on the inside of the needle curvature. The effective cutting edges are restricted to the front section of the needle and merge into a triangulated body which continues for half the length of the needle.

A Unique Needle Range

Needles	**Advantages**
Blunt point needle	Improving safety
Taper point	Gentle separation of fibrous tissue
BV needle	Consistancy pass after pass
Visi-black needle	Visibility is their strength
Cc needle	Easy penetration of calcified coronary
Hemo-seal	Needle suture fitting choice for vascular surgery
Multicurve needle	For confined access procedure
Taper cut needles	Easy penetration of dense tough tissue
Prime needle	Excellence in skin closure

Advanced Needle Coating

Advanced needle coating technology provides a new level of smoothness during tissue penetration.

Advantages

- Maintains needle sharpness from start to finish over multiple pass
- Offers consistant needle penetration pass after pass and needle-to-needle
- Enhances needle control and placement
- Covers entire needle tip to swage for consistently smooth passage through tissue.

Needle Shapes

The choice of needle shape is frequently governed by the accessibility of the tissue to be sutured, and normally, the more confined the operative site, the greater the curvature required. The basic shapes involved are as follows: ¼, 3/8, ½, 5/8, J shape, compound curved, straight.

CHAPTER

13

Arterial Cannula

IDEAL CHARACTERISTICS OF ARTERIAL CANNULAE

An ideal cannula should have all these characteristics:

- Ease of insertion
- Predictability of flow
- Minimal size/maximum flow capability
- Flexibility.

Selection Criteria

Surgeon must choose the appropriate size and shape of cannula according to patient's BSA and type of surgery.

Size of Cannula

- Measured by unit French (3 Fr)—Indicates the radius of the outside diameter of the cannula tip 3 Fr = 1 mm
- Blood flow depends on size and wall thickness of cannulae
- Goal is to select the narrowest bore cannula that will deliver expected flow without causing excessive turbulence at pressure gradient not greater than 100 mm Hg.
- Size ranges from 6 Fr to 24 Fr.

TYPES OF CANNULAE

- Each cannula has unique design
- Structure, tip, body, differ

- Commonly used cannulas with
  - Straight tip
  - Curved tip
  - Angled tip—45°, 80° (plastic, metal tip available).

Features

Wire-reinforced	With flange	With side holes	With vented connector
Non wire-reinforced	Without flange	Without side holes	With non-vented connector

Side Holes

Use of cannula with side holes may reduce pressure gradients, reduce jetting and turbulence.

Flanges

Flanges in cannulas aid in fixation and prevent too deep insertion into aorta; use of a short aortic cannula with a flange may prevent insertion into brachiocephalic artery.

Wire Reinforcement

Prevention of kinking and twisting of cannula.

Tip Orientation Line

Line on cannula indicates direction of beak. Beak is directed towards middle of transverse arch to avoid entering arch vessels.

Vent-Connector

It helps in de-airing during priming of the cannula.

STRAIGHT TIP ARTERIAL CANNULA (NONWIRE INFORCED)

- Feature beveled, thin wall tips attached to tapered cannula bodies (Fig. 13.1)

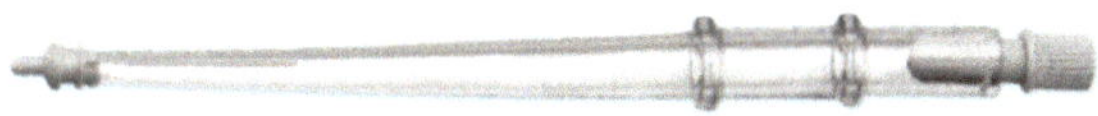

Fig. 13.1: Straight tip arterial cannula chonwire inforced

- Available in pediatric and adult sizes
- A tip orientation line permits precise positioning of the cannulae.

Advantages

- Flexible design
- Both adult and pediatric sizes
- **Tip orientation line**—Line on cannula indicates direction of beak. Beak is directed towards middle of transverse arch to avoid entering arch vessels.

Disadvantage

- Short length
- Chance of kinking.

STRAIGHT TIP (WIRE REINFORCED)

- Elective cardiac surgeries for short-term bypass
- Wire reinforced prevents kinking (Fig. 13.2).

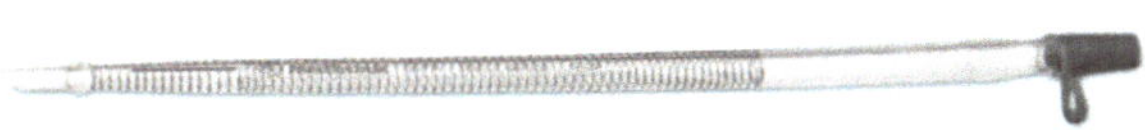

Fig. 13.2: Straight tip (wire reinforced) cannula

Disadvantage

If cannula not placed properly it can—

- Damage posterior aortic wall
- Dislodge atheroemboli (sand blasting)
- Cause arterial dissections
- Disturb flow into nearby vessels.

PEDIATRIC ONE-PIECE ARTERIAL CANNULAE

- Straight tip, elongated, one piece, kink resistant, wire bound bodies (Fig. 13.3)

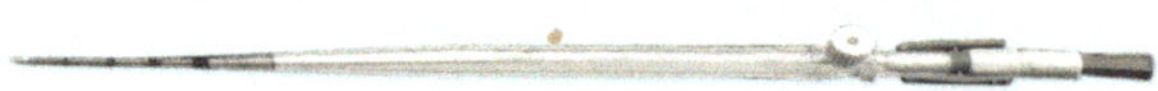

Fig. 13.3: Pediatric one-piece arterial cannula

- Adjustable flow—guard style introducer along with depth markings permit precise positioning of the cannulae.

Advantage

- Optimizing access within the sternotomy space on even the smallest pediatric patient
- Exclusive flow-guard features provide hemostasis while priming the cannulae.

Disadvantage

- Accidental direction of cannulae tip towards branch arteries of aortic arch
- Increased intracranial blood pressure.

FLEXIBLE ARCH CANNULAE

- Beveled tip with tapered one-piece bodies
- Adjustable depth ring with tip orientation and depth markings (Fig. 13.4)

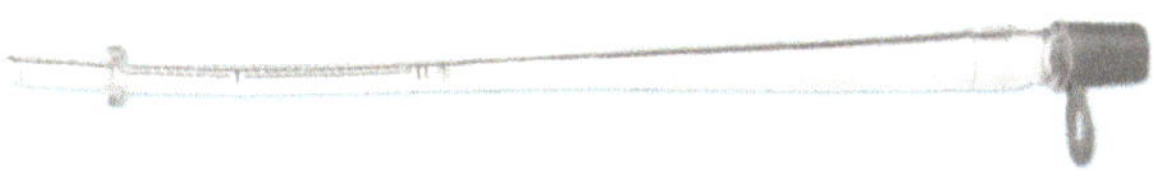

Fig. 13.4: Flexible arch cannula

- **Use:** Used mainly in arch repair surgeries, redo surgeries.

Advantage

- Flexible design provides easy positioning of cannulae on the incision site
- Depth ring on the cannulae aid in fixation to prevent too deep insertion into aorta.

Disadvantage

- Available in adult size only
- Kinking possible because of flexible body.

ANGLED TIP ARTERIAL CANNULA

- Beveled, thin wall tips with tapered, one piece, kink resistant wire bound bodies
- Higher flow rates with minimum pressure difference
- Tip orientation line available.

Advantage

- Tip point towards arch rather than towards wall of aorta, less damage to vessel wall

- Positions the connection site further away from the surgical field
- Side holes help diffuse and disperse blood flow, results in reduced jetting and turbulence.

Disadvantage

- Chance of diverting more emboli from clamp region towards the upper vessels.

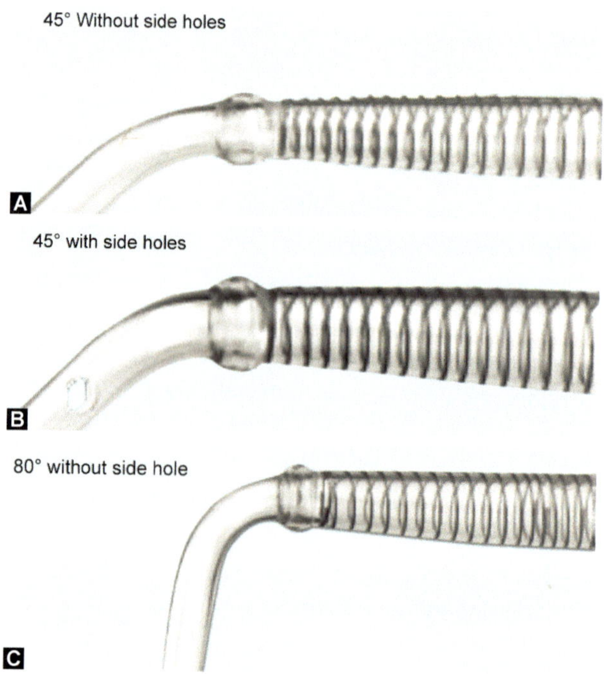

Figs 13.5A to C: Angled tip arterial cannula. (A) 45° without side hole; (B) 45° with side hole; (C) 80° without side hole

CURVED TIP AORTIC CANNULAE (WIRE INFORCED)

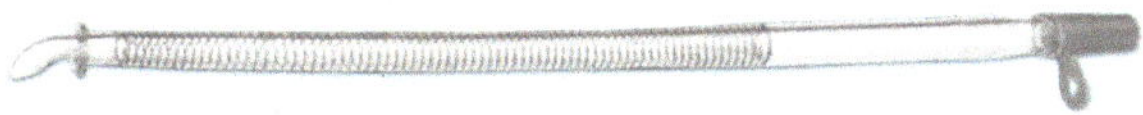

Fig. 13.6: Curved tip aortic cannula

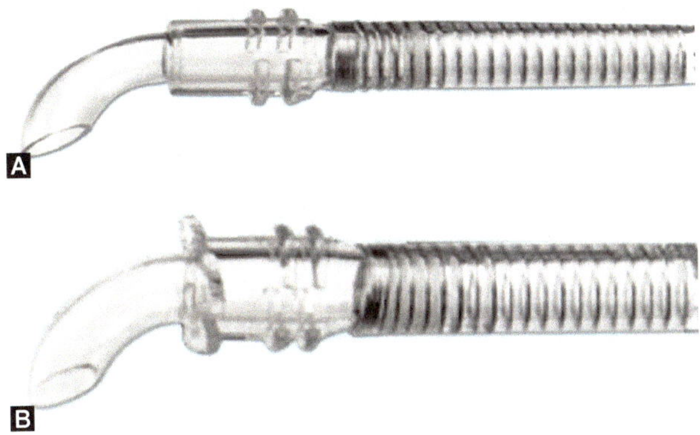

Figs 13.7A and B: Curved tip aortic cannula. (A) Without flange; (B) With flange

Advantage

- Flanges in cannulas aid in fixation and prevent too deep insertion into aorta; use of a short aortic cannulae with a flange may prevent insertion into brachiocephalic arteries
- Less shear stress on aortic wall
- Reduced risk of dislodging emboli to cerebral vessels.

Disadvantage

- Stronger jet flow
- Higher shear stress inside the cannulae
- Highly distributed flow, more stagnant near clamp region.

METAL TIP ARTERIAL CANNULAE

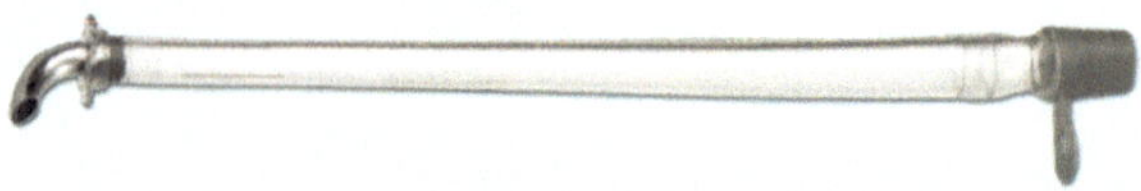

Figs 13.8: Metal tip arterial cannula

- Beveled, thin wall, curved metal tips attached to tapered cannula bodies
- Construction allows for higher flow rates with minimal pressure differential
- Choice of either standard or soft flange are available
- Tip orientation line permit precise positioning of the cannulae.

Advantages

- Metal tips confirm to the shape of the aorta to improve positioning and stability.

Disadvantage

- Increased trauma to aortic tissue wall because of metal tip
- Increased jetting effect and turbulence of blood
- High chance of microemboli, hemolysis
- Can be used for adult patient only.

ELONGTED ONE-PIECE ARTERIAL CANNULAE (STRAIGHT)

Special Features

- Elongated one piece arterial cannula (Fig. 13.9)
- Thin wall tips kink resistant wire wound bodies

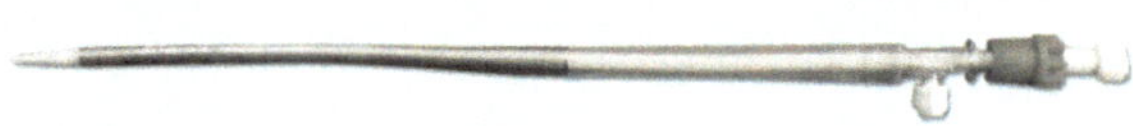

Figs 13.9: Elongated one-piece arterial cannula

- Introducer along with depth markings, radiopaque suture collar permits precise positioning of cannula
- Introducer—blunt, dilator tip.

Use

- Can be used for both femoral, aortic cannulation
- Used in arch repair, aortic dissection surgeries.

Advantages

Reinforcement wire allows considerable flexibility without kinking.

Mainly used in trans-apical approach of cannulation of aorta as an alternative of other sites because of its elongated tip.

Disadvantage

Not available in smaller sizes for use in pediatric patient.

Forceful insertion of guide wire can cause trauma or dissection of aorta.

EOPA CAP ARTERIAL CANNULA

Special Feature

- Thin wall tips with elongated, one piece, kink resistant wire-wound bodies (Fig. 13.10)
- Have an integrated pressure monitoring port

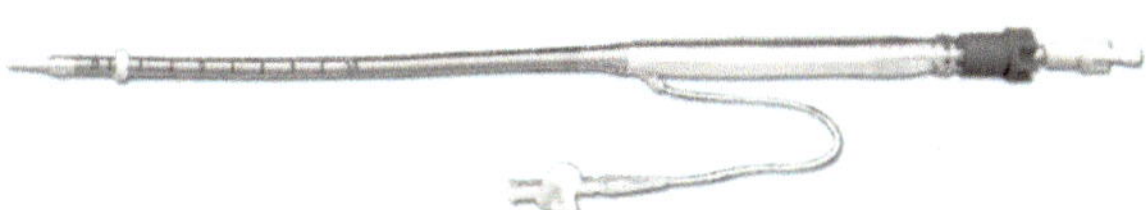

Fig. 13.10: EOPA cap arterial cannula

- Real-time display of accurate central arterial pressure
- Dilator along with depth marking, radiopaque suture collar permit precise positioning of cannula.

Advantage

- Separate integrated pressure lumen with 3 way stopcock
- Accurate pressure information provides the ability to better adjust CPB flow
- Eliminate the need to pave a pressure needle in aorta.

Disadvantage

- Chance of accidental air emboli through pressure port 3 way.

OPTI-SITE ARTERIAL CANNULAE

Features

- Design to accomodate multiple surgical techniques and clinician preferences (Fig. 13.11)
- A lock feature reduces push back of the introducer during insertion
- Vent cap reduces back-blood when no guidewire is used in procedure
- Depth markings aid in placement.

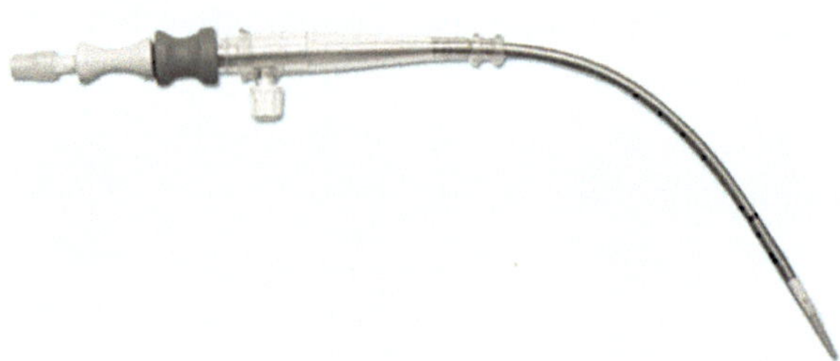

Fig. 13.11: Opti-site arterial cannula

Advantage

Allows safe insertion for additional arterial access sites, such as aorta, axillary, subclavian arteries.
Size available: 16–22 Fr.

Disadvantage

- High chances of kinking due to ultra thin wall design.

EMBOL–X–GLIDE PROTECTION CANNULAE

- Most efficient intra-aortic filtration device available, filter is integrated with the cannula (Fig. 13.12)
- Low trauma out flow path with advanced filter technology because of dispersion
- Central orientation of the cannula tip is designed to reduce direct jetting of flow against the aortic wall.

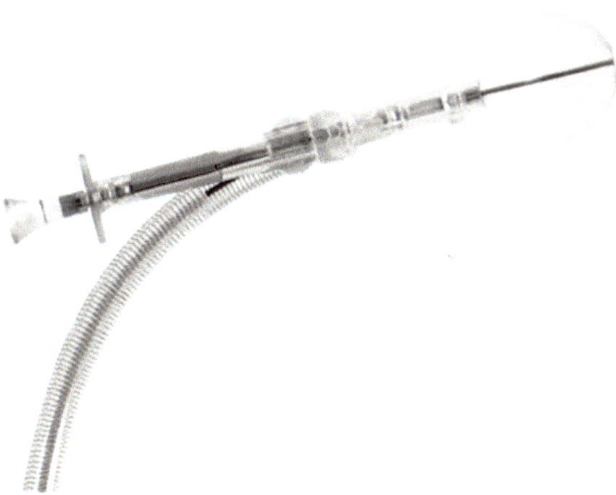

Fig. 13.12: Embol-X-glide protection cannula

Advantages

- Advanced filter technology demonstrated to provide safe and effective emboli capture, reduction of adverse neurologic and end organ events
- Specially designed autodilating tip requires only a small incision
- Filter integrated in to a conventional cannula design for ease of use
- Not only captures particulate matter in bloodstream, also helps reduce risk of particulate matter released by return flow to aorta.

Disadvantage

- Failure or block of integrated filter can happen very rarely.

CHAPTER

14

Venous Cannulae

- Venous cannulation is performed to drain and divert the venous return of patient to the CPB system
- Venous cannulae have to be selected according to the surgical plan whether caval (or) bicaval cannulation is needed.

TYPES OF CANNULAE

- Venous cannulas vary according to their structure, tips, length.

STRUCTURE

- RGID, malleable
- Single stage, two stage, three stage
- Straight tip, right angle tip
- Right angle tip has plastic end, metal tip
- Tip design is varied:
  - Light house tip
  - Open light house tip
  - Bullet tip
  - Pilot tip
  - Open basket, closed basket.

TWO-STAGE VENOUS CANNULAE

This cannula is designed in such a way that tip of cannula can drain IVC while body part drain right atrium (Fig. 14.1).

Features

- Flexible cannula body
- Wire wound kink resistant construction
- Available in low profile, oval body design to provide more room in the surgical field
- Additional depth mark allows shallow placement for assisted venous drainage
- Multiport light house tip with enlarged end hole for added drainage.

Uses

This cannula is mainly used for:

- On pump CABG
- Aortic valve replacement.

Designs

Three designs of body are available:

- Reduced stage body—29/37 Fr
- Thin wall body—29/29 Fr
- Oval body—32/40, 36/46, 34/46, 36/51, 28/36.

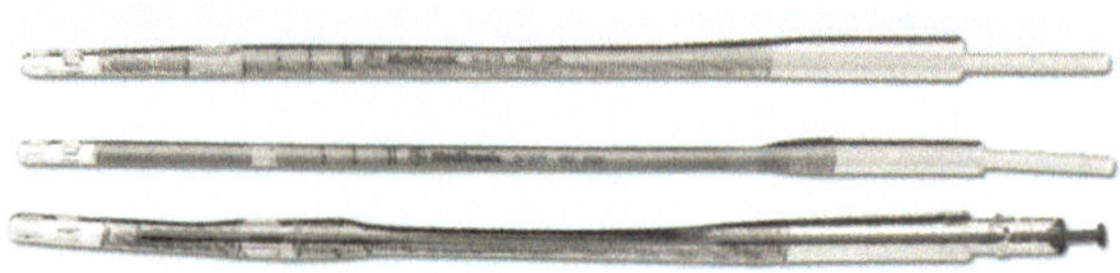

Fig. 14.1: Two-stage venous cannulae

VC2™ ATRIAL CAVAL VENOUS CANNULAE

Features

- Non-wirewound body, wire wound body, oval wire wound body (Fig. 14.2)
- Patented swirl tip and large slotted atrial basket minimizes flow restriction
- Atraumatic and flexible swirl tip designed to promote ease of insertion and to sustain an open channel through vena cava during surgery.

Advantages

- Soft pliable swirl tip promotes continuous flow and minimizes chatter
- Unique oval body permits cannula to be positioned away from the surgical field
- Swirl tip provides increased atrial drainage and offers an uninterrupted pathway for venous return from IVC.

Size

- Nonwire wound body—34/51 Fr
- Wire wound body—34/38 Fr, 34/48 Fr
- Oval wire wound body—34/38 Fr, 34/48 Fr.

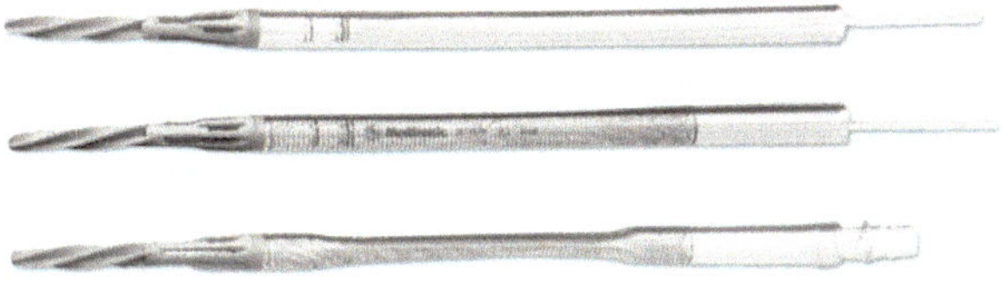

Fig. 14.2: VC2™ atrial caval venous cannulae

ULTRAFLEX VENOUS CANNULA

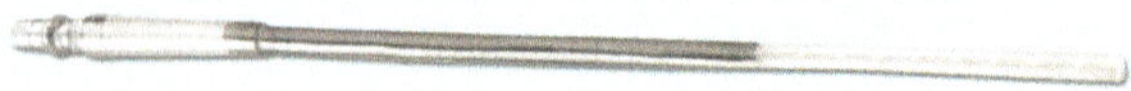

Fig. 14.3: Ultraflex venous cannula

Features

- Polyurethane, thin walled, wire-wound body
- Unique uni-stage tip, depth markings, radiopaque stripes, multiple side holes at the distal tip (Fig. 14.3)
- Malleable stylet within the cannula obturator aids in introduction and positioning of cannula
- Thirty two cat-eye shaped holes in the tip reduces kinking
- Open lighthouse tip with enlarged end hole minimizes the potential for line chatter
- Ridges running between 2nd and 3rd stage openings, channel and maintain blood flow during collapse or emptying of RA
- Size: 29/29/29 Fr.

VAD CANNULA—FOR VENTRICULAR ASSIST

- Suited for left or right atrial cannulation (Fig. 14.4)
- Kink resistant, wire wound body
- Radiopaque, right angle, swirl tip.

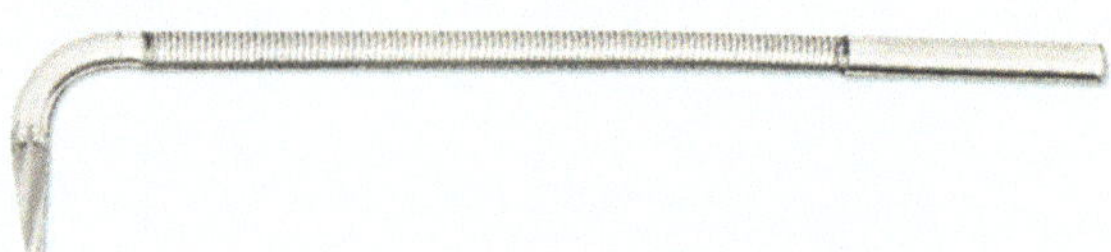

Fig. 14.4: Cannula for ventricular assist

Advantages

- This design maximizes continuous venous drainage flow rates from atrium and minimizes collapsing around the tip
- Size: 36 Fr.

SINGLE STAGE CANNULA WITH BASKET TIP

- Features nonwire wound body with an atrial basket
- Design maximizes venous drainage flow rates (Fig. 14.5).

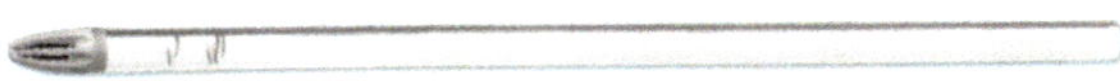

Fig. 14.5: Single stage cannula with basket tip

SILICONE SINGLE STAGE VENOUS CANNULA WITH INFLATABLE CUFF

- Bicaval cannula features silicone, kink resistant wire wound body with an inflatable cuff (Fig. 14.6)
- Size: 37 Fr.

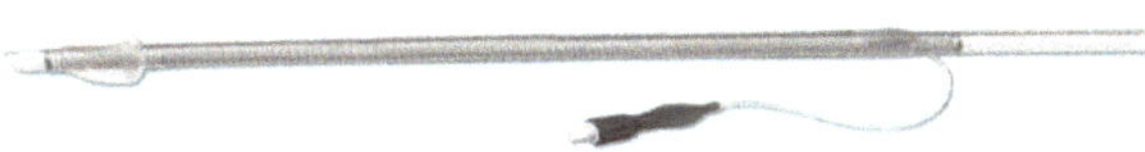

Fig. 14.6: Single stage cannula with inflatable cuff

MALLEABLE SINGLE-STAGE VENOUS CANNULAE

Features

- Malleable one piece kink resistant, wire wound bodies with tapered, multiport tips (Fig. 14.7)
- Integrates malleable wire outside the wire winding to optimize internal diameter for maximum flow performance

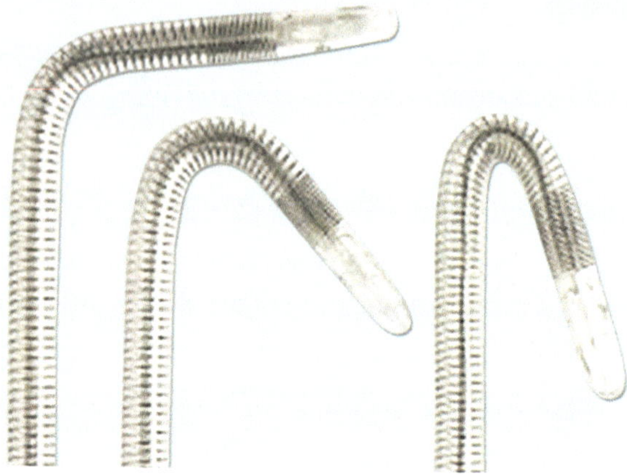

Fig. 14.7: Malleable single-stage venous cannulae

- Depth marks allow for tip manipulation and gauging of insertion depth during use
- Flow performance equals to nonmalleable models.

Advantages

- Ability to vary length of cannula from bends to tip to best fit surgeon preference
- Can be customized to the anatomy of the patient
- Ability to create a wide range of bend angles in order to minimize cannula torque in RA.

Bending Procedure

- Cannula will maintain the desired angle best when bent to the left or right while depth marks and malleable wire are facing the person handling.
- Size available: 12–40 Fr.

SINGLE STAGE VENOUS CANNULA

- Used for Bicaval venous drainage for cannulating SVC and IVC separately (Fig. 14.8)
- One piece, kink resistant, wire wound body
- Thin wall PVC construction
- Tapered multiport bullet tips for easy insertion
- Depth markings permit precise positioning
- Size: 12–40 Fr.

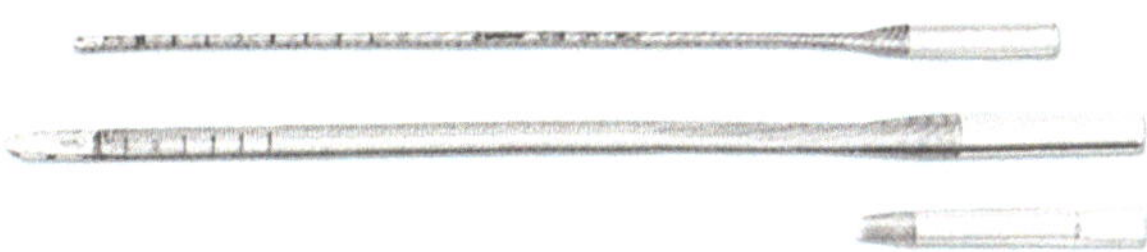

Fig. 14.8: Single-stage venous cannulae

SINGLE STAGE RIGHT ANGLE VENOUS CANNULA

- One piece, kink resistant, wire wound body (Fig. 14.9)
- Right angle bent end with tapered multiport bullet tip
- Thin wall PVC construction
- Depth markings permit precise positioning
- Size: 12–40 Fr.

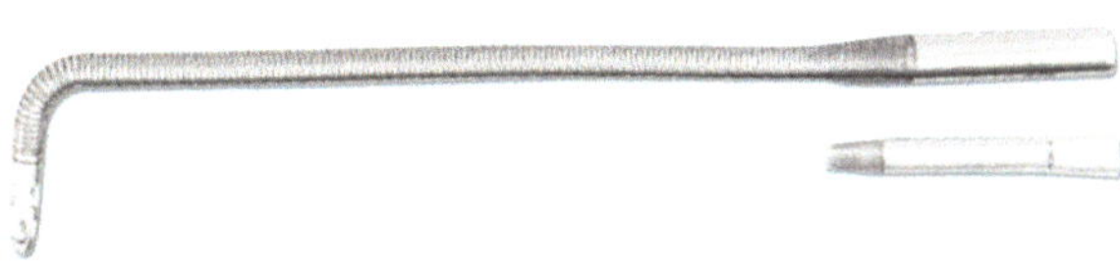

Fig. 14.9: Single-stage right angle venous cannulae

RIGHT ANGLE METAL TIP VENOUS CANNULAE

Features

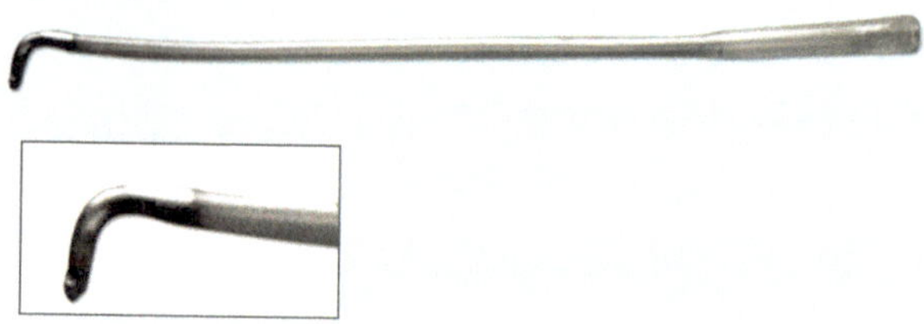

Fig. 14.10: Single-stage metal tip cannulae

- Ultra-thin 0.016 inch metal wall construction bodies (Fig. 14.10)
- Flexible, kink-resistant wire wound cannula bodies
- Thin walled beveled tip and side port design maximizes flow rate
- Tip orientation line permits precise positioning of the cannulae
- Available in standard tip and extended tip length.

Advantages

- Metal tips facilitate insertion and hold lesser chances of malpositioning
- Provides maximum ID to OD ratio less affected by heart rotation.

Disadvantage

- Tissue trauma may happen due to forceful insertion
- Right a lower case Angle plastic tip cannula also available.

CHAPTER

15

Vent and Sump Catheters

- Vent catheters are designed to empty the chambers of heart, thereby providing a cleaner operative field and minimizing the possibility of air embolism
- Vent catheter prevents over-distension of cardiac chamber during CPB.

LEFT HEART VENT CATHETER

- These vent catheters are for direct and indirect venting of LV and feature perforated tips
- Choice of either PVC or silicone with straight, preformed and malleable body with depth markings (Fig. 15.1) is available
- Straight body come with a malleable or stiff guidewire style introducer for easy insertion and placement
- Pediatric and adult sizes 10, 13, 16, 20 Fr
- Bullet tip and right angle features facilitate insertion

Fig. 15.1: Left heart vent catheter

- Depth markings
- Guidewire stylet available on certain models
- ¼ vented (or) nonvented slip connector.

MALLEABLE LV VENT

- Pediatric and adult sizes 10, 13, 15, 16, 18, 20 fr
- Malleable wire in tip (or) full length
- Malleable wire permits precise shaping and ¼ connector (Fig. 15.2).

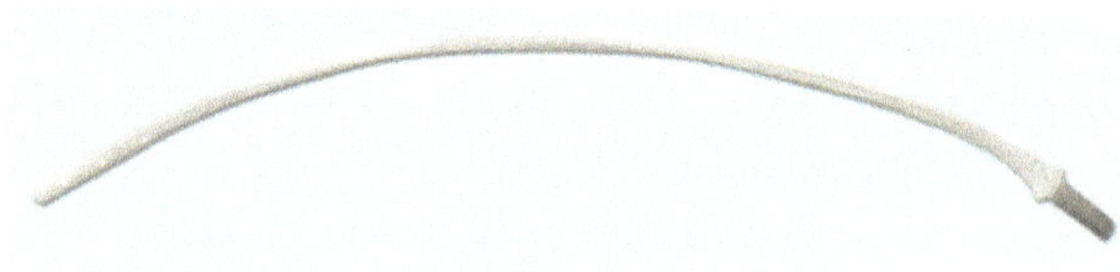

Fig. 15.2: Malleable LV Vent

Disadvantage

- Degree of suction should be monitored to reduce the possibility of air embolism.

PULMONARY ARTERY VENT CANNULA

- Used to empty the left atrium via the pulmonary vasculature
- Soft pliable tip with 12 side holes
- Movable collar
- Introducer needle for easy introduction and placement
- 1/4"threaded
- Movable depth marker.

AORTIC AIR ASPIRATING NEEDLE

- Needle features 16 ga (5 fr) stainless steel needle with two side slots and flange (Fig. 15.3)

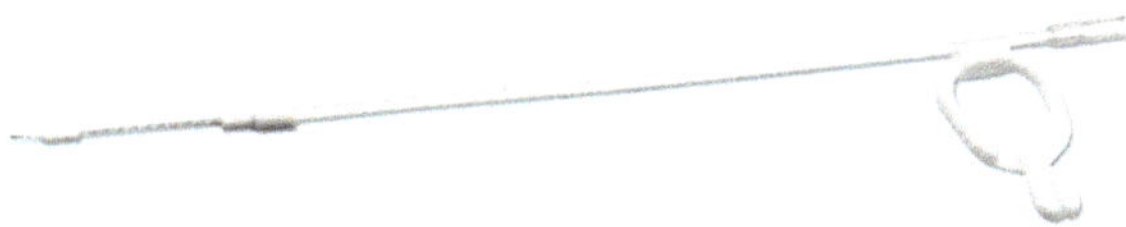

Fig. 15.3: Aortic air aspirating needle

- Soft, flexile PVC tubing
- Roberts clamps
- ¼"connector
- Perfect for aspirating air from ascending aorta.

SUMP CATHETERS

Features

- Multiport venting tips for optimal suction
- Mayo-style sumps are available with or without a metal weight in the tip
- All sump style may be used with the phrenic nerve pad in the pericardium.

PERICARDIAL SUMPS

- Feature a fluted tip which is encased in a stainless steel spring, has a weight at the end
- Spring wound for optimal suction
- Tip is attached to soft flexible tubing terminating in slip connector
- Weighted tip facilitates positioning in pericardial waddle
- 1/4"and 1/8"connector available.

Disadvantage

- Pericardial sump models are not indicated to be placed through a valve to drain a closed cardiac chamber as it can suck leaflet or chordate.

INTRACARDIAC/PERICARDIAL SUMP

- Versatile design for both intracardiac and pericardial use
- Weighted perforated pool tip to maximize suction and minimize tissue trauma
- Mayo-style tip allows atraumatic intracardiac use
- Perforated tip is attached to tubing, ends with ¼"slip connector
- Size—20 Fr.

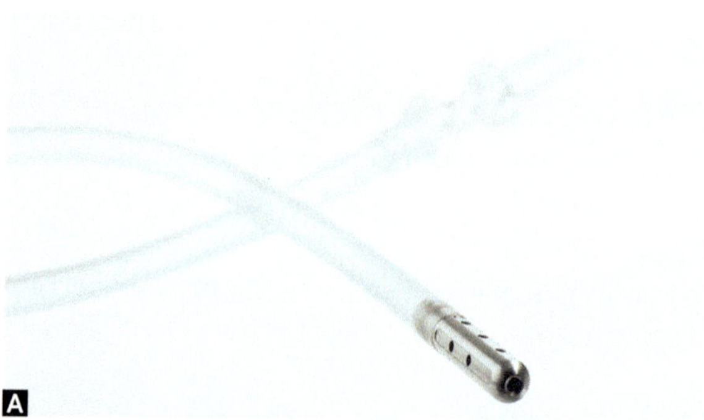

A

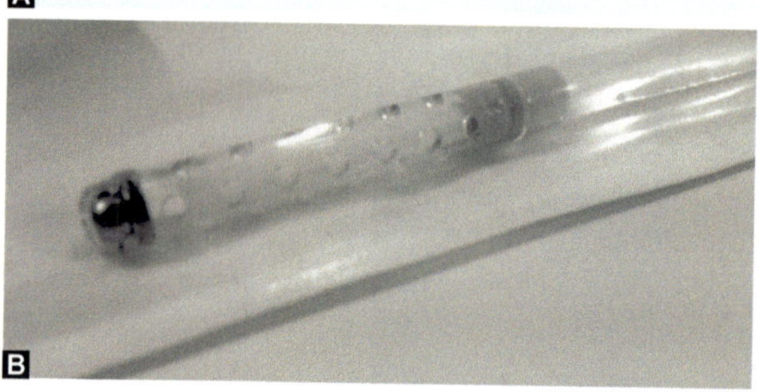

B

Figs 15.4A and B: Pericardial sump

INTRACARDIAC SUMP

- Perforated pool tip to maximize suction and minimize tissue trauma
- Multi-port vent tip atraumatic to internal chamber structures
- ¼"connector
- Adult size (20 Fr) and pediatric size (12 Fr) available.

CARDIAC SUCTION TUBES

- Cardiac suction tubes are designed to remove blood and other fluid from surgical site
- Provides a clearer operative field and prevents excessive pooled blood in chest cavity
- Features several hand grip and tip options to support a variety of suction use techniques.

MALLEABLE CARDIAC SUCTION TUBES

- Features pencil hand grips with a vacuum control port
- Tip shaft is made from malleable stainless steel that can be shaped to surgeon's preference
- Available with or without a soft silicone tip
- Equipped with a length of tubing and clamp terminating with ¼"(0.64 cm) slip connector.

Tip Models

- Soft tip, Olive tip, Frazier tip
- Size: 6 Fr, 10 Fr.

INTRACARDIAC SUCTION TUBE

- Pencil hand grip with malleable stainless steel shaft
- Perforated pool tip to maximize suction and minimize tissue trauma
- Size: 10 Fr, 20 Fr.

RIGID SUCTION TUBES

- Features comfortable hand grip
- Tip shaft is made from rigid stainless steel
- Macrosucker has fluted tip to maximize suction and minimize tissue trauma
- Mini-sucker has a soft, vented tip designed to clear blood from anastomotic site with gentle suction
- Terminate in ¼"barbed connector.
- Size: 16 Fr, 20 Fr.

CHAPTER

16

Cardioplegia Cannula

- Cardioplegia is delivered to arrest the heart to facilitate bloodless field for visualization during surgery and also provides myocardial protection to heart during arrest
- Cardioplegia can be delivered through:
  - Antegrade—aortic root
  - Retrograde—through coronary sinus
  - Coronary ostia—directly into coronary arteries.
- Different types of cardioplegia cannulas are available according to the surgical needs.

AORTIC ROOT CANNULA

Features

- Used to infuse cardioplegia into the aortic root or to aspirate air from the aorta (Fig. 16.1)

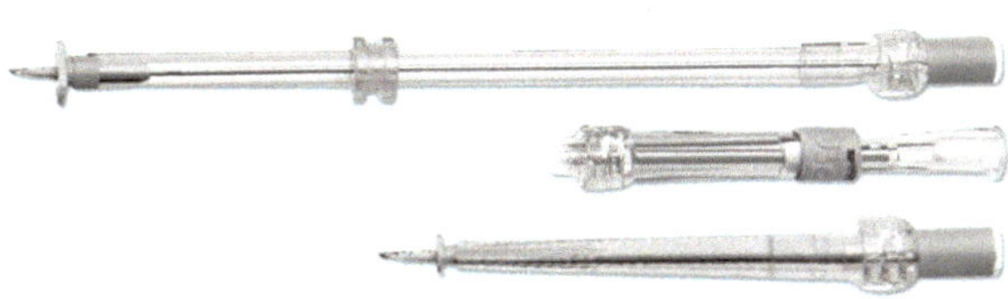

Fig. 16.1: Aortic root cannulae

- Length of cannula is designed to allow connection to the CP circuit outside the chest cavity
- Flanged collar provides a predetermined insertion depth and also aids in securing the cannula
- Large bore cannula body provides high flow rates
- Integral suture rings aid helps fix cannula
- All cannula are supplied with a stainless steel introducer needle.

Advantages

- Radiopaque tips attached to clear body
- Available in standard tip, long tip, pressure monitoring tip.

AORTIC ROOT CANNULA WITH LONG TIP

Use

In minimal invasive surgery and cardiac surgery through thoracotomy (Fig. 16.2).

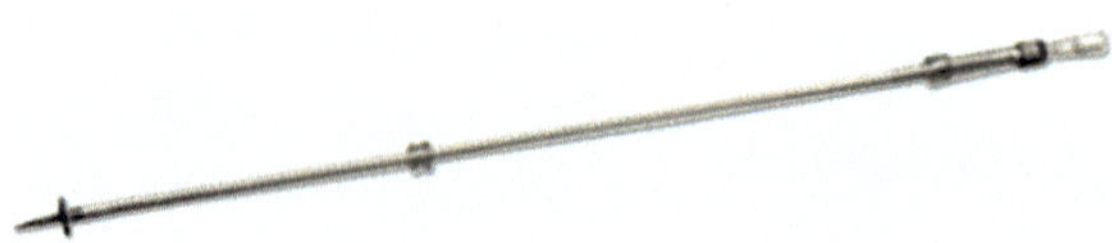

Fig. 16.2: Aortic root cannulae with long tip

AORTIC ROOT CANNULA WITH PRESSURE MONITORING TIP

- Design enables the monitoring of actual aortic root pressure while infusing cardioplegia
- Also available with attached vent line allowing venting of left heart, delivery of cardioplegia, monitoring of aortic root pressure all via single device.

AORTIC ROOT CANNULA WITH VENT LINE

- Has all features of original aortic root cannula with addition of vent line
- Administration of cardiolplegia and left heart venting can be done with same cannula (Fig. 16.3).

DUAL-LUMEN AORTIC ROOT CANNULA

- Used for simultaneous infusion of cardioplegia solution and aspiration of air from the aorta (Fig. 16.4)
- Reduces possibility of introducing air into the coronary artery bed
- Subsequent infusion of cardioplegia solution without having to clear the line of air possible.

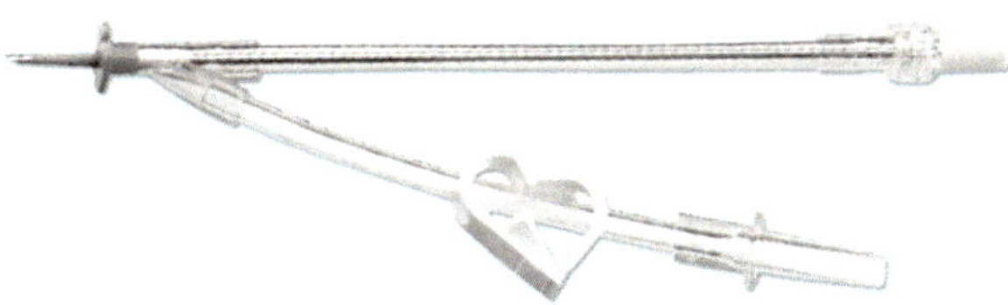

Fig. 16.3: Aortic root cannulae with vent line

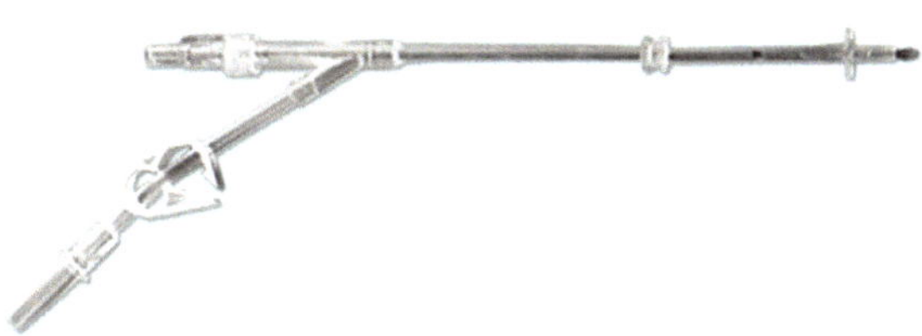

Fig. 16.4: Dual-lumen aortic cannulae

PEDIATRIC AORTIC ROOT CANNULA

- Available in 18 ga (4 Fr) tip to meet needs of pediatric patients (Fig. 16.5)

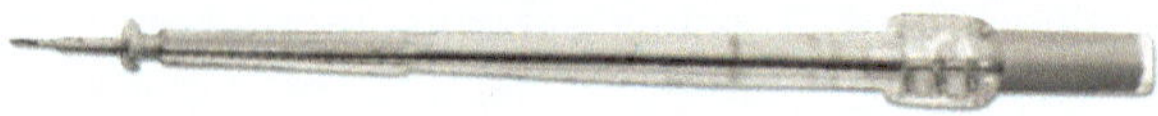

Fig. 16.5: Pediatric aortic cannulae

- Has ribs on cannula body to prevent kinking.

AORTIC ROOT CANNULAE WITH FLOW-GUARD INTRODUCER

- A flow-guard system allows retraction of needle point into a rigid fitting after cannula is placed (Fig. 16.6)
- Reduces possibility of accidental punctures
- Features an introducer needle for controlled priming that can be retracted without loss of blood from the cannula.

CORONARY OSTIAL CANNULA

- Used to deliver cardioplegia directly through coronary ostia
- Available in two unique designs:
  - Basket tip
  - Soft tip.

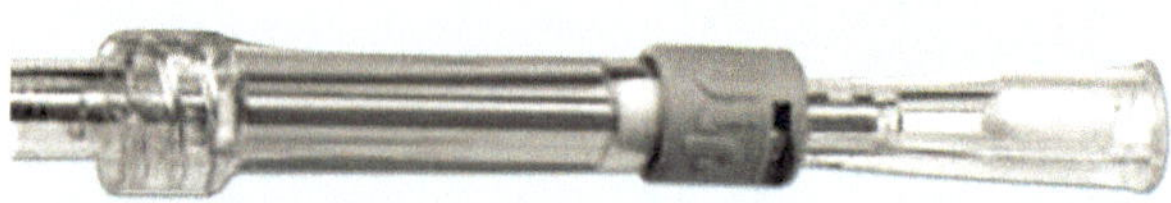

Fig. 16.6: Aortic root cannula with flow guard introducer

Basket Tip Style

- Soft radiopaque plastic basket tip with soft flange to occlude ostium to prevent backflow of cardioplegia (Fig. 16.7)

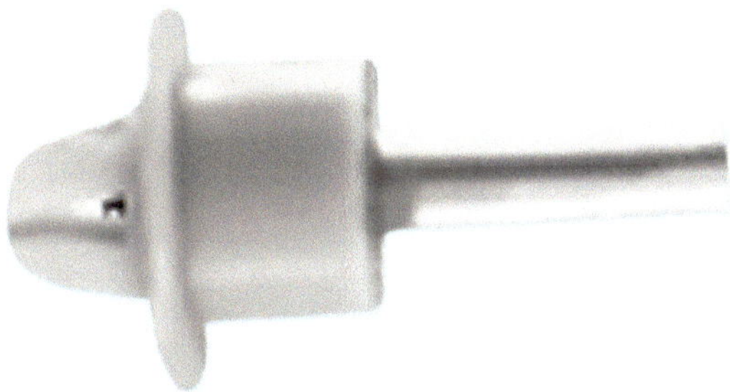

Fig. 16.7: Basket tip style coronary ostial cannula

- Light weight construction with a locking female luer end
- Malleable stainless steel shaft can be shaped to most appropriate angle
- Also available with extra-wide flange, provide an even better seal around the coronary ostia

45° Coronary Ostial Cannula (Basket Tip)

- High flow cannula
- 45° Soft flanged tip with a malleable shaft (Figs 16.8A and B)
- Comfortable handle permits easy tip manipulation

90° (Coronary Ostial Cannula Basket Tip)

- High flow cannula
- Soft, flanged basket tips
- Malleable Shafts allow user to preform cannulae to most functional shape
- Comfortable handle permit easy tip manipulation
- Large bore metal tubing allows greater flow at lower pressure

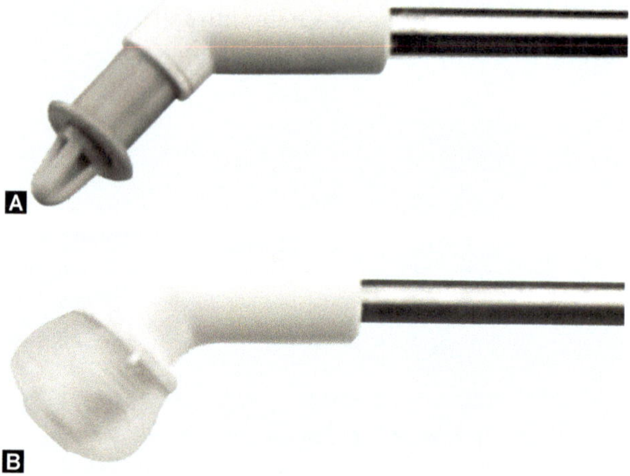

Figs 16.8A and B: 45° Coronary ostial cannula (basket tip)

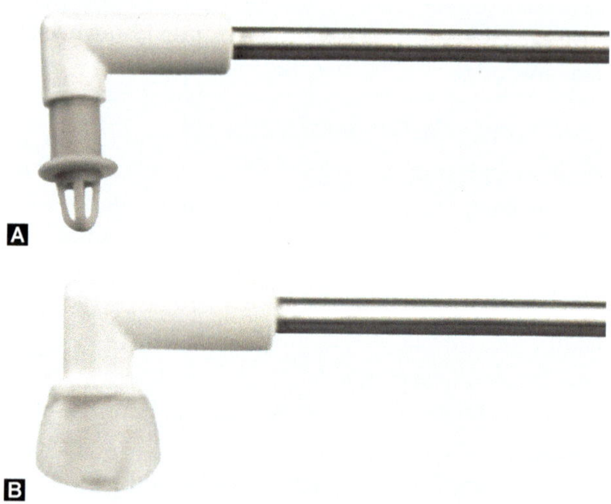

Figs 16.9A and B: 90° (Coronary ostial cannula basket tip)

Soft-tip Style

- Silicone gel-filled tip seals snugly around ostium (outside) without trauma to the intima
- One size can accommodate various sizes of coronary arteries
- Malleable shaft can be shaped to any angle for either left or right coronary (Fig. 16.10)

90°and 45° Coronary Ostial Cannula (Soft Tip)

- High flow cannula (Figs 16.11A and B).

Silicone Coronary Artery Ostial Cannula

- Soft bulb provides a tight seal around coronary ostia to prevent backflow of cardioplegia solution (Fig. 16.12)

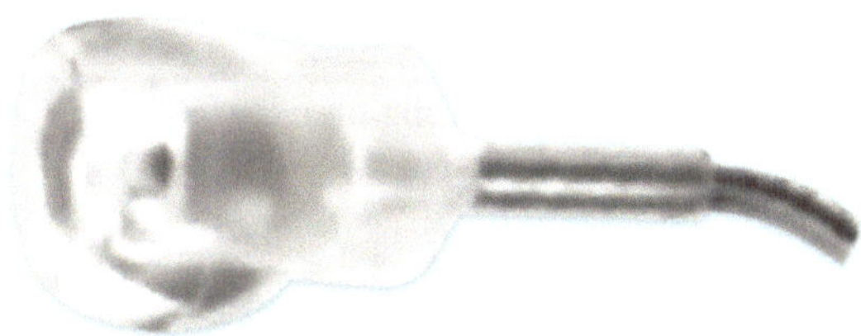

Fig. 16.10: Soft-tip style coronary aortic cannula

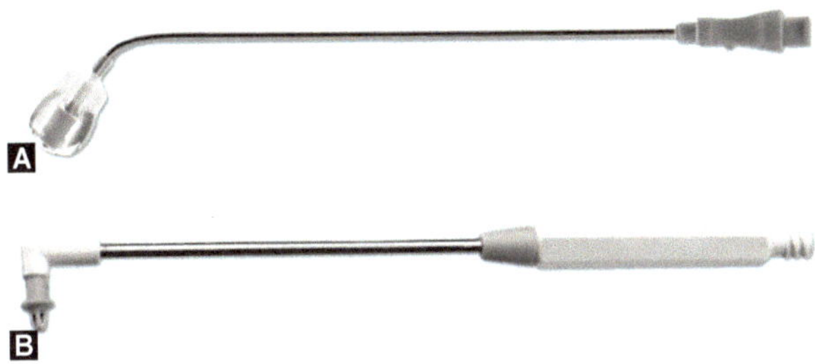

Figs 16.11A and B: 90° and 45° Coronary ostial cannula (soft tip)

- Silicone body provides flexibility during hypothermic cardioplegia delivery.

RETROGRADE PERFUSION CANNULA

- Silicone RCSP cannulae with manual inflate cuffs
- Silicone body, manual inflate cuffs with pressure monitoring lines with integral stop lock
- Solid stylet or guidewire stylet with true-touch handle available
- Syringe for cuff inflation present.

Types of Cuff

- Smooth cuff—easy placement
- Performed cuff
- Ridged cuff—enhanced retention
- Cuff can be standard or elongated.

Advantage of Elongated Cuff

- Standard coronary sinus perfusion techniques allow a portion of retrograde cardioplegia to be shunted away from capillary vessel through middle cardiac vein
- Cannula with elongated balloon to block the middle cardiac vein, shunting is avoided, cardioplegia is directed to capillary beds providing uniform myocardial protection.

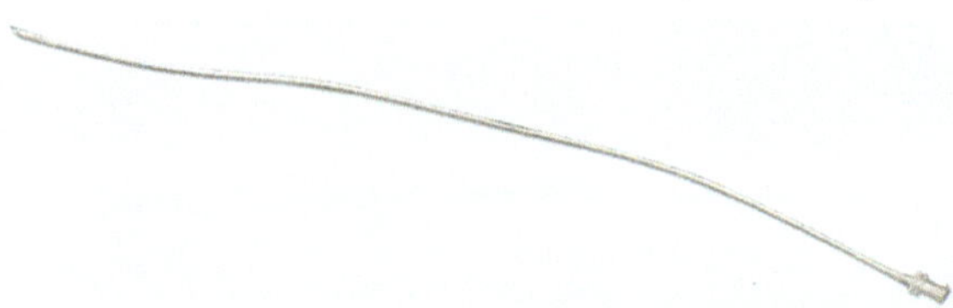

Fig. 16.12: Silicone coronary artery ostial cannula

SILICONE RCSP CANNULAE WITH AUTO INFLATE CUFF

- Cuff inflation without need of syringe
- Unique flow through design allows cardioplegia to circulate through the cuff before exiting the cannula tip
- Cuffs also feature dual pressure monitoring system (Fig. 16.13).

Advantage

- Normally provides intra-sinus pressure through integral port in the tip
- If the tip is inadvertently occluded, the second port will monitor intracuff pressure this reduces the coronary sinus rupture due to over inflation
- Tips: 6, 10, 13, 15 Fr.

BALLOON CUFFS

- Manual inflate (silicone)
- Auto-inflate (silicone or polyurethane)
- Smooth for easy placement or ridged for enhanced retention

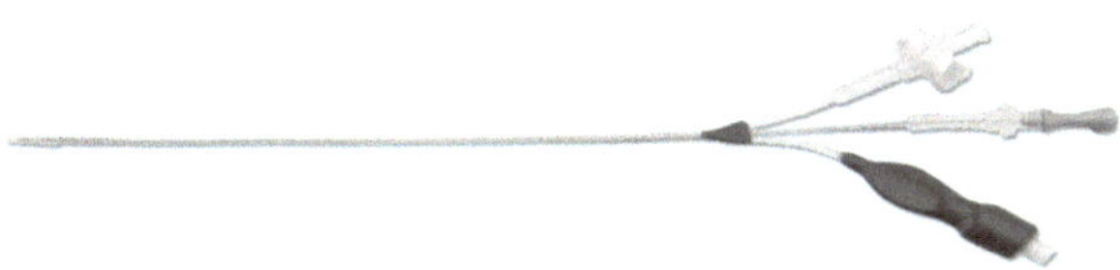

Fig. 16.13: Silicone RCSP cannula with inflate cuff

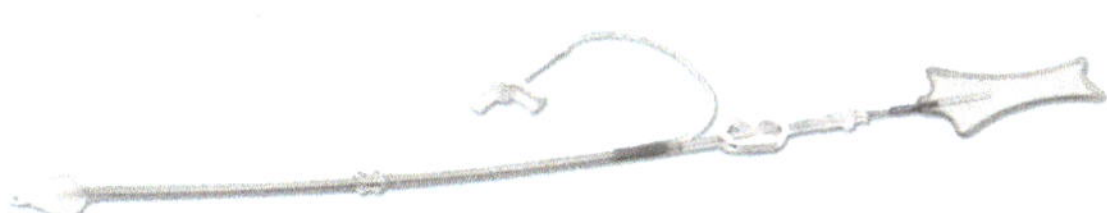

Fig. 16.14: DLP PVC RCSP cannula-auto inflate

- Standard size or elongated for enhanced retention and occlusion of middle cardiac vein.

Body

- Soft silicone for flexibility
- PVC for enhanced controls.

Stylet

- Malleable guidewire stylet
- Solid stylet for firmer control.

DLP PVC RCSP CANNULA-AUTO INFLATE

- PVC bodies
- Polyurethane autoinflate cuff with integral pressure monitoring line
- Available in smooth and ridged preformed cuff with multiport tip, short fluted tip (Fig. 16.14).

Index

Page numbers followed by *f* refer to figure and *t* refer to table.

D

E

F

G

H

I

J

K

L

M

N

O

P

R

S